Praise for *How Can You NOT Laugh at a Time Like This?*

"While writing a great book on how to recover from illness, Carla Ulbrich wrote an even better book on how to live a healthy and fulfilling life. No doubt, you have a good doctor if you see *How Can You NOT Laugh at a Time Like This?* in their waiting room."

—Michael Stock, WLRN Radio

"*How Can You NOT Laugh at a Time Like This?* is outstanding. . . . Carla is your guide to navigate the often emotionally and technically confusing world of illness with heart, humor, and bite-size chapters. Everyone needs a patient advocate—and now you have one, with this book!"

—Robert Aubry Davis and Mary Sue Twohy, "The Village," Sirius XM Radio

"As a doctor, Patch Adams brought to mainstream America the concept of a caring, compassionate, and fun medical staff making a profound difference in the healing of their patients. Now we've been given the gift to hear about it from the patient's perspective. Carla Ulbrich is living proof that bringing fun, play, creativity, and laughter to the healing process does wonders for the mind, body, and spirit. Carla's uncanny wit is infectious—and that's an infection we can all benefit from!"

—Danny Donuts, CPA (comic perform̶a̶n̶c̶e̶ ̶a̶r̶tist) and member of the Assoc̶i̶ Humor

"I was completely taken̶ ̶ ̶ ̶ ̶ ̶ ̶ok on life, her tenacity, and ĺ̶ ̶ ̶ ̶ ̶ nestly, on every level, in̶ ̶ ̶ ̶ ̶ ̶ ̶ ̶tastic ̶ ̶ ̶ ̶ ̶ ̶mor."

—LuckyYogini.com

How Can You NOT Laugh at a Time Like This?

Reclaim Your Health with Humor, Creativity, and Grit

Carla Ulbrich
(The Singing Patient)

tell me
New Haven, Connecticut

Back cover photo © Jayne Toohey
Illustrations by Ted Enik

Library of Congress Control Number 2010936321
ISBN: 978-0-9816453-4-6 (softcover)
ISBN: 978-0-9829421-4-7 (e-book)

Printed in the United States of America
First edition
10 9 8 7 6 5 4 3 2 1

Published by **Tell Me Press**, LLC
98 Mansfield St.
New Haven, CT 06511
www.tell**me**press.com

Editorial director: Lisa Clyde Nielsen
Art direction, text and cover design: Linda Loiewski
Editing: Justine Rathbun
Proofreading: Anita Oliva
Production and marketing: Jeff Breuler, Jeff Eyrich, Traci Crampton
Publicity: Susannah Greenberg

Contents

Chapter 1
It's Not as Fun as It Looks: Other People and Your Disease

Chapter 2
What's Up, Doc? Surviving Health Care

Chapter 3
That's Inflammatory! What Not to Eat If You Have an Autoimmune Disease

Chapter 4
Well, Duh! Science Proves Common Sense Right

Chapter 5
Rubber Chicken Soup: Keeping a Sense of Humor

Chapter 6
Take a Mind off Your Load: Expressing Yourself and Keeping It Positive

Chapter 7
I'd Like to Speak to the Owner of This Body: Moving Forward and Taking Responsibility

Chapter 8
The Early Bird Can Have the Worm: Pacing Yourself

Chapter 9
Mirror, Mirror, on the Wall, Who's the . . . Oh, Never Mind: Beauty

Chapter 10
Mission Possible: Persistence

Acknowledgments

A big thank-you to Ruth Williams Hunsinger, who came up with the idea of "three faces," and to Fibro UK, a support group that came up with the phrase "Fibromyalgia: the other *F* word."

Thanks also to my very patient husband, muse, and best friend, Joe Giacoio; cheerleader and sage Emry Gweldig; my parents, Carl and Holley Ulbrich; Easy the nurse dog; friend and fellow funny lady Deirdre Flint; friend and confidant Grant Livingston; friend and host Dave Cambest; friend and unofficial personal nurse Laurie McDonough; "extra parents" Joan and Richard Sheinwald and Bob and Saralyn Singer; my co-counselors, especially Judy; my healers, especially Dava Michelson, Janet Galipo, Janet Parker, and Adam Frent, DO; everyone who saw past my illness to the real me; and those who believed in my potential to get completely better. Or if they didn't, they never let me know it. And for those who thought I was nuts and said so, well you just made me more determined, so I thank you, too.

• • •

Introduction: Play This Song Backward; or How I Became the Singing Patient

I'm a performing songwriter. I write about everything from Klingons to Waffle House. Some say my songs are funny. Some just find them laughable. But for the past fifteen years I've managed to eke out a living with my wacky songs. When people ask me why in the world I turned out so strange, I trace it back to interactions with people like my grandmother.

I always enjoyed making my grandmother laugh, because then she'd quit asking me when I was going to get married. And because I could make her laugh, I got away with saying the most outrageous things. When she was trying to find something to wear to a wedding, I said, "Well, Gram, you know what they say: if you can't wear something nice, don't wear anything at all." People can't stay mad at you if you can make them laugh.

I spent the first two and a half decades of my life making people laugh, playing all kinds of musical instruments, flirting with boys, and spending many beautiful South Carolina days on my bike, in a pool, or at the lake. I was so strong that even though I was barely five feet tall, I played the tuba in the marching band. (They called me "the tuba with legs.") I was writing songs even back then, including a few funny ones, although I never shared them with anyone.

But when I got seriously ill at age twenty-five, I lost my sense of humor for a while. It took two years to get a diagnosis, and while I was waiting for that to happen, I kept getting sicker and sicker—my hair fell out, I had fevers spiking to 104°F every day, and the illness cost me my job and savings. At my literal lowest, I weighed eighty pounds, could not get out of a chair by myself, and hadn't eaten an actual meal in probably two months. Turns out I was suffering from several autoimmune diseases, one of which was causing my kidneys to fail.

Autoimmune disease is what happens when your immune system starts attacking your healthy tissues; it can't tell self from nonself. Of my several diagnosed disorders, lupus was the most life-threatening. Its symptoms range from mildly annoying (rashes) to devastating (kidney failure). Mainstream medicine has no idea what causes this process of self-destruction and offers no cure, instead attempting to control symptoms with powerful, sometimes toxic drugs. Progressive doctors and alternative medicine practitioners, I later learned, believe it is caused by multiple factors, and they offer a much sunnier prognosis—if you're willing to work really hard at wellness.

Don't get me wrong: the path to wellness isn't straightforward, and fighting a chronic illness sometimes feels like "one step forward, two steps back." As my health improved, I started to pursue my dreams of teaching guitar, writing songs, and performing local gigs—I was reaping the rewards that come with regained health. Then I hit roadblocks, such as experiencing two strokes and facing kidney failure again. But I refused to believe that I would have anything less than a full recovery. Hope itself is powerful; so long as there's hope, there's hope. I completely recovered from the strokes, and eight years later, I still have my kidneys. They work just fine.

Illness can touch your life in unexpected ways. When I was in college, I had crippling stage fright. I wrote lots of songs, and I would sign up for open mikes and talent shows but run away before the emcees called my name. A funny thing happens when you face kidney failure and chronic disease and overcome them: you have a lot to sing about, and the stage isn't so scary anymore. And that's how I became the Singing Patient.

This book is the result of my years of searching for—and finding—better solutions than mainstream medicine had to offer by itself. I didn't abandon mainstream medicine, but I didn't end my search there, either. I didn't want to "manage" my disease with drugs for the rest of my life. I wanted to be healthy again. Today I don't have all the answers, but I do have my original kidneys, and I'm doing better than predicted and taking only one prescription (for high blood pressure).

My remissions did not happen by chance; I worked hard for them. I had to do some soul searching and take responsibility for what I ate, how I exercised, how I spent my time, and who I hung out with. I learned that having a sense of humor is essential to health. But I didn't do anything anyone else couldn't do, assuming they knew where to start.

There's an old joke: What do you get when you play a country song backward? You get your truck back, you get your wife back, you get your dog back. . . . Well, I wrote some songs about my medical journey, and even though they're not country and I've never played them backward, I got my hair back, I got my kidneys back, and I got my sense of humor back. If your health is not perfect, here's the good news: you can get better. Maybe just a little better. Maybe a lot better. Maybe completely better. Most of all, I hope you join me in finding laughter in both the good times and the tough—truly, how can we not laugh at a time like this?

What seems nasty, painful, evil can become a source of beauty, joy, and strength, if faced with an open mind.

—Henry Miller

• • •

Chapter 1

It's Not as Fun as It Looks: Other People and Your Disease

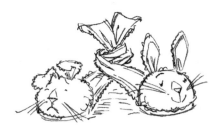

Top Ten Annoying Things to Say to Someone Who's Just Been Diagnosed

Hate and fear can poison the body as well as toxic chemicals.
—Joseph Krimsky, MD

Nobody plans to walk into someone's hospital room and blurt out insensitive, inappropriate comments. And yet it happens all the time. If Hallmark had a section for "This is going to hurt you more than it hurts me," the following phrases would possibly be the top ten best sellers. (And in case you are caught unprepared, I'm including my responses—feel free to steal them or improvise your own!)

Inappropriate comments: when silence isn't awkward enough.

10. *"I knew someone who had that. She died."*
    (Thanks for the boost of confidence!)

9. *"I know someone who has that; he's in perfect health."*
    (You can't be in perfect health when you've been diagnosed with a serious illness.)

8. *"Is that a form of cancer?"*

   (Ask a doctor, or look it up on the Internet. The appropriate response is not curiosity but compassion.)

7. *"Is that a form of AIDS?"*

   (See comment 8, above.)

6. *"God is punishing you because you have a hidden sin in your life." Or: "The devil is attacking you because you are doing God's work."*

   (Mr. Wizard, Don Knotts, the founder of the Peace Corps, and two serial killers were all diagnosed with cancer. Disease is not doled out on a "who deserves this most?" basis.)

5. *"I'm sure it's nothing. You'll be fine."*

   (Great! I'll cancel all my doctor appointments.)

4. *"Is it genetic?"*

   (If you're not my twin, why does that matter right now?)

3. *"Have you tried [insert any form of alternative medicine you can think of here]?"*

   (There's time for problem solving later. Be a friend first.)

2. *"You don't look sick."*

   (You don't look insensitive. I guess appearances can be deceiving.)

And the number-one annoying reaction to a diagnosis of serious illness:

1. *"Is it CONTAGIOUS?!"*

   (Yes! And you can't leave until I LICK YOUR FACE!)

When I've been the visitor, I'm sure I said something less than perfect. I truly understand now why police are instructed to always say to the victim's family, "I'm sorry for your loss." Better to sound like a prerecorded message than to blurt out something idiotic.

Here's what I wish folks would say:

- "You don't have to be brave."

- "I've been thinking of you."

- "I'm sorry."

- "Can I bring you something?" (Some of my favorite gifts when I'm in the hospital: a tabletop fan, a pillow, my favorite stuffed animal, something to read, my iPod, food that doesn't taste like cardboard, a funny movie, meditational CDs, a notebook to draw or write in. Thoughtful gifts for someone with lupus, Raynaud's, or fibromyalgia who is out of the hospital: a heating pad, a Pampered Chef jar opener, a paraffin wax hand bath, hand and foot warmers, a Backnobber self-massager.)

- "I don't know what to say."

- "I am praying for you. We are all praying for you."

- "What can I do for you?"

- "How can I help?"

- "Let's do something fun as soon as you're feeling better."

- "I'm here for you."

- "Don't worry about answering all those phone calls and e-mails. People understand you're not up to it right now."

- "I'm checking in on your house and your cat twice a day."

- "I have a cold so I stayed home rather than risking infecting you." (Thank you!)

Even as we deal with much pain, fear, anxiety, and uncertainty as patients, those around us are also dealing with a lot of emotions. It's a shock to see someone you care about weak and helpless. Our friends and family feel helpless, too, and afraid. People want to help—they just don't know what to do. If we give people something to do or say, they won't feel so helpless, and we won't feel so neglected. It won't stop everyone from saying stupid things, but maybe it'll be a little less annoying if I'm holding my favorite stuffed animal, reading *Calvin and Hobbes*, and eating some chocolate.

• • •

Sometimes It Is Better to Receive

They say what doesn't kill you makes you stronger. Then it kills you. I'm not afraid of death. However, I, like most people, am afraid of suffering. I'm even more afraid of suffering alone, and this is why some sort of human connection is so important when you're ill.

One of the most memorable (in a good way) moments from my hospital stays lasted only a few minutes. One evening a worker, not even a nurse, came by when I was upset. I had just been told I would be getting chemotherapy that would leave me sterile and would also be getting transfusions and high doses of prednisone. I was pretty freaked out. This kind person saw me in distress, sat down, and sang to me and held my hand.

She wasn't there more than three minutes probably, but it sustained me for days. I have no idea who she was. For all I know, she was an angel. Whoever she was, she put aside her own agenda, her own fears, and her own problems for a moment and changed my world for the better.

Other gestures I will never forget were the nurse who brought me pudding after I slept through dinner and the time my friend Laurie snuck in some food for me when I was in the hospital all day waiting for a transfusion. (The doctor hadn't written a diet order, so the staff wasn't allowed to feed me.) Laurie was wonderful company, and she took me to some of my appointments when I wasn't allowed to drive (doctor's orders; not a commentary on my driving record).

A songwriter I barely knew named Grant Livingston visited me twice in the hospital, after which we became good friends. When I couldn't play the guitar due to my symptoms, he learned all the guitar parts to my songs so I could still sing them in concert.

I was fortunate to have such generous people cross my path, but it was not always the case. In my first twelve years of having a chronic illness, I had no significant romantic relationships, and for about five of those years, I lived alone. During those years I had little to no help, and I was partly to blame. I was so proud that I was independent—a little too proud—that when someone did offer help, I always refused. I couldn't even receive a compliment gracefully.

I had to learn to ask for what I need. That does not come naturally to me. I'd rather pretend I have no needs at all. (Of course, pretending I have no needs may have had something to do with my getting into this mess in the first place.) I also had to learn to accept help. At some point I realized that if I continued to refuse help, not only would I make things harder on myself, I would deprive someone else the pleasure and satisfaction of feeling they made a difference. Not coincidentally, once I allowed people to help me, I had a lot more help. Huh. Finally, I learned to say no—to too many activities, to too many visitors, and to spending time with "psychic vampires" (people who drain you emotionally)—and say yes to people who truly cared.

I thought I would rather die than speak up for myself. The thing is, now that my health is stable, I probably won't die anytime soon—but if I don't get my needs met, I could just barely hang on for decades, suffering. I would definitely rather speak up for myself than suffer. If I learn to do that, then what didn't kill me will definitely make me stronger.

• • •

Angels with Fur

I read somewhere that a doctor spending thirty seconds by a patient's bedside is equivalent to standing in the doorway half-engaged for fifteen minutes. Just being there, really being there, even for only a moment or two in a day, to say, "I see you. I hear you. I do not judge you. I'm here for you" is so helpful. You don't need to have answers. Listening is enough.

You know who are really good at being there? Animals. I'm thankful I had a cat when I was first diagnosed. His name was Slick. He was funny, smart, mischievous, and a lap cat. I adopted him shortly before I got sick and had him for about nine years. He used to sleep in bed with me until I moved into my mom and dad's house. (Maybe he felt self-conscious, not being married and sleeping together under my parents' roof.)

One day I went to the doctor and found out I had had a stroke. The following night I was terrified. Since the stroke had happened while I was asleep, I was afraid to go to sleep again. About 3:00 a.m., I heard a scratch at the bedroom door. It was Slick. Somehow, from an entirely different part of the house, he knew I needed him. He jumped into bed with me and stayed there until I got up late the next day. He didn't even get up for breakfast (and he loved food).

Now my husband and I have a Maltese dog named Easy. She's a nurse, clown, empath, and angel all rolled into one. She stays with me in bed, no matter how long I sleep. When I was alone and sick, I did not take good care of Slick. (I wasn't doing such a hot job of taking care of myself.) But as long as I am in a situation where someone else can make sure the pet is cared for if I can't do it, I will always have a pet in my life. Pets always treat me the same, whether I look good or bad, whether I am able to work or not, whether I am sad or happy.

Some hospitals offer visits from therapy dogs or cats—you may need to ask for this service specifically. And for those institutions that don't offer pet therapy, sometimes you can get permission to have a pet brought in to visit you. I managed to bring my dog to see my aunt in the hospital. It's not as complicated as you might think to arrange such a visit, and it's well worth the effort.

• • •

Disease Envy

I'm always baffled when people are envious of my health struggle.

I lost a lot of weight when I was sick—food was repulsive to me. I was so thin that I had no butt. I had to carry a cushion with me everywhere because it hurt to sit. Someone had the nerve to say to me, "I wish I'd lose my appetite." What did I wish I'd said? "I'll swap you a stroke and kidney failure for a big butt!"

Someone else said to me, "I wish I could just lay around in the bed and read." You know, it's okay to have the thought—just don't say it out loud. If your life is so miserable that you're envious of someone who's just been diagnosed with a debilitating illness, maybe it's time to make a few life adjustments.

Once I heard someone refer to envy as an inner compass. The desire to have what someone else possesses points you in the right direction. So rather than let that somewhat healthy emotion—envy—simmer and turn into resentment, which is toxic, we should pay attention when we feel envy and say to ourselves, "What is it that this person has in his life that I'm lacking in mine?" Upon reflection, you might realize that you don't really want a stroke or kidney failure; you just need a little "me" time or some attention from a loved one. Meanwhile, it's okay to have the envious thought—just don't share it with me.

"On the Commode Again"
(Sing to the tune of "On the Road Again")

On the commode again

I can't believe I'm on the commode again

Some people call it makin' music with a rear end

And I can't believe I'm on the commode again

On the commode again

Goin' in places that I've never been

Seein' things I hope I never see again

And I can't believe I'm on the commode again

• • •

You Look Fine

You do not determine your success by comparing yourself to others, rather you determine your success by comparing your accomplishments to your capabilities.

—Zig Ziglar

Have you ever told someone about your diagnosis only to have him say to you, "You look fine"?

Maybe it's supposed to be a compliment. But then why do I want to scream? Probably because in that context what I hear is "I don't believe you." You can't see an autoimmune disease, so how do you know by looking at people how healthy they are? Besides, maybe you're only seeing the sick person on one of their few good days, the ones when they are up, dressed, made up, and out and about. (On the other hand, I'm glad I don't always look as bad as I feel. If I did, I'd have long periods of being butt ugly and wouldn't want to see anyone. But it does create a mental hurdle for folks who can't believe what they can't see.)

It reminds me of how we look at other people's relationships and think, "Oh, their marriage is perfect." Then we're stunned when they split up. It's never smart to compare your inner experience with someone else's outer appearance. After all, whenever reporters interview the neighbors of a serial killer, the neighbors always say, "He seemed so nice." We just don't know what's really going on behind closed doors and between other people's ears.

If you want to take it upon yourself to educate someone, you can order pamphlets from the support group particular to your disease. There are societies for most illnesses that provide this kind of informational support. But if you're tired, or if you feel your words will fall on deaf ears, you can always answer a "You look fine" with a twist on the words of Billy Crystal: "It is better to feel good than to look good, darling."

• • •

Lessons from the Nudist Festival: How Much to Reveal

One of the venues on the acoustic-music circuit is a nudist festival in West Virginia. I've played there several times and always enjoy it. Clothing is optional, and, yes, I always take the clothing option.

The first time I played there, I marveled at the courageous men grilling hot dogs and using staple guns in the nude. Then I had to get used to being onstage, looking out and seeing an audience of naked people. Suddenly, that nerve-calming strategy of imagining the audience in their underwear gained new meaning. And urgency.

Then I sat down and had dinner with some of the folks. Now, the "offending parts" were all below table level, and I realized that these nudists were intelligent, interesting people. It was *my* hang-ups about nudity that made me uncomfortable; the issue was mine, not theirs.

I'd chosen to enter the sanctuary of their inner circle, and I knew going in that they would be naked. I had no grounds for being offended by their choices (they were just nude—they weren't having sex in the open). They didn't demand that I remove my clothes, and I didn't demand that they put theirs on.

When these folks leave the colony, they put on clothes. They don't try to make the nudity thing work everywhere they go. They blend with the norms of society when they are out in it. It's not worth the punishment to try to make the rest of the world understand their point of view.

What could this possibly have to do with having a serious illness? More than meets the naked eye.

The nudist colony, a safe place where everyone is a nudist, is like a support group where everyone is struggling with an illness. In the safety of the support group we can "let it all hang out," be ourselves, and not worry about being judged. If someone comes to the meeting and isn't sick, he would be really out of line to shout, "Hey! Can't we talk about something besides illness and feelings? How 'bout those Giants?"

When we leave the safety of the support group, we have a choice: we can remain "nude," wearing our feelings and problems on our sleeve and talking constantly about our illness, or we can choose to "put on clothes" and try to blend in with the rest of society.

"It's not fair!" you shout. "I have a right to talk about my illness. It's bad enough I'm sick, and now I have to worry about other people not being able to handle it?"

You can talk about your illness as nakedly as you want, as long as you are willing to accept the consequences. Just like nudity, some folks are going to have issues with your being sick, not necessarily because of your own hang-ups about being sick, but because of *their* hang-ups about being *around* someone who is sick. It forces them to think about mortality, their own vulnerability, or the fairness of the universe, when they'd much rather be out on the beach building a sand castle and believing illness and death could never happen to them. It's going to stir up fear, and that's going to make some people say and do hurtful things. This includes family, who have their own very strong emotions about their loved one being ill.

Decide how much of yourself you want to expose. The "clothing" is not really to protect others, it's to protect you. Rather than try to turn the rest of the world into the compassionate people you wish they were, realize their limitations, stop trying to get blood from a stone, and divulge the gory details only to those who can handle it. Choose your listeners wisely.

Having a devastating illness comes with lots of powerful emotions that need to go somewhere, however. Find yourself a "nudist colony" of safe people where you can be honest about your illness and feelings without getting punished for it. This can be in the form of a healthy support group, where feelings are handled in a compassionate manner. If you can't find a good one nearby, start one or join one online. And you always have the sacred secret space of your diary or journal, where you can say anything and everything you need to express.

Then, you can put your clothes back on and join the rest of the world, where you can talk about something besides your illness and forget your troubles for a bit. At some point it's going to be a welcome relief to hear "How 'bout those Giants?" instead of "How are your kidneys?"

How much should you reveal to the world? That's up to you. A thong? A burka? Something in between? Totally nude? It is your choice, at all times, to choose when and to whom you reveal your illness and the details about it.

Here's how I handle it. When I'm among other patients, or performing at a health conference, or in other safe environments, I speak about my illness openly. No one in these settings is bothered by such talk, and we have helpful, meaningful conversations. But I'm well aware that out in public—at dinner parties or hanging with friends—folks don't want to hear about that sort of thing for the most part. So I don't impose it on them, and I don't open myself up to being hurt by their fears or ignorance.

If someone asks me how I'm doing, I give a short summary. I'm not dishonest about my symptoms or my well-being, but I don't usually tell people my diagnosis. Sometimes I just answer, "Good, thanks for asking," or "Been a little tired, but I'm doing okay," or sometimes I'll put in a good word for acupuncture or whatever else I'm doing that's working for me.

If I know the person a lot better, I give a bit more detail, but I don't feel the need to go on for long in a social gathering, because I have other, safer outlets for my emotions, and I don't want "unsafe" people to overhear too much and start asking invasive questions. There's a time and a place to be naked.

• • •

It's Never Lupus. Except When It's Lupus

On the TV series *House, MD*, the fictitious Dr. House told all of America (and Britain) that "It's not lupus. It's never lupus." If you're dealing with lupus, that's the last thing you need to hear.

For millions of people around the globe, it is lupus. All day, every day, it's freaking lupus. Pain, fatigue, even organ failure and death. Hearing "It's never lupus" is a slap in the face. On top of that, the comment seems to be confusing the medical community. Almost every time I see a new specialist, they don't believe me when I tell them I have lupus. They say things like "Who told you that you have lupus?" and "I don't usually believe that diagnosis." Then they run their own battery of tests, only to later march back into the room and announce to me that I have lupus. Oh, gee, really?

Look, I don't want lupus. I wish I didn't have lupus. And I hope one day I can say I no longer have lupus. If I were going to choose a disease to pretend to have, I'd pick one with more cachet. One that people take seriously. Like, well, pretty much anything other than lupus.

What I really don't understand is why anyone thinks this so-called running joke is funny. Would it still be funny if the fictional TV doc was saying "It's never MS" or "It's never cerebral palsy" or "It's never an aneurysm"? Of course not. And yet, somehow, "It's never lupus" is acceptable. Why? Because the word lupus sounds funny? I say we rename the disease to something horrible sounding, like, oh, I don't know, long, slow agonizing death syndrome.

Thanks to the dedication of volunteers and the patronage of some celebrities, the perceptions of some diseases have moved past their former stigma and are now talked about openly and with compassion. Why does one disease inspire people to run a marathon, while another disease inspires a running joke? Lupus not only lacks its own celebrity spokesperson, it's the only disease I can think of that has an antiawareness campaign. Which is why, in my fantasy series finale of *House, MD,* the House character develops lupus.

• • •

Chapter 2

What's Up, Doc?
Surviving Health Care

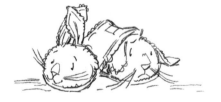

So, You Come Here Often?

Ever stop and think about how bizarre the doctor-patient relationship is? Within five minutes of meeting you, the doctor knows your age, weight, and any embarrassing ailments in your or your family's history. And you're in your underwear. And you don't even know his first name.

Imagine being in any other setting and being asked these questions by a total stranger. If you were on a blind date, he wouldn't make it past the server bringing the ice water.

"Hi, nice to meet you. Let's see, now . . . how old are you?" (*slap!*) "What do you weigh?" (*slap!*) "Any pregnancies?" (*slap!*) "When was your last period?" (*slap! slap!*) "Are you sexually active?" (*punch!*)

But there you are in the doctor's office, and while you're talking the doc jots down various things on his clipboard: white female, 120 pounds, age twenty-nine (okay, I'm lying a little bit), nonsmoker, nondrinker, scar on left side. Sounds like a personal ad. (Well, until the scar part. Then it sounds like you're describing someone who just robbed a liquor store.)

If you were describing yourself to someone you were actually trying to get to know, you'd mention something about your personality and beliefs, maybe even your religious preference. If a doctor ever asks me my religious preference, I know it's not because he's trying to get to know me as a person—it's because he's about to do something to me that increases my chances of meeting Jesus face-to-face. Soon.

It's too bad doctors have to rush through appointments and don't have a chance to get to know their patients as people, because taking time can give some insight into what may have brought on their ailment. Plus getting to know folks can be a real treat. I love sharing conversation with new acquaintances: finding common ground, hearing about their hobbies, learning where they're from. Doctors don't have time for all that; they have to cut to the chase. They typically only have eight minutes per patient. (Most of my dates lasted at least twice that long.)

So, I wondered, how can we make the most of these eight minutes? I had an opportunity to sit across a table and converse with Dr. Patch Adams, so I asked him, "How do I get my doctor to treat me more like a human being?" This is what he said:

There is plenty of pain to go around. Not only are the patients suffering, the doctors, nurses, and administrators are all suffering from an abusive, oppressive system that sucks the meaning and joy out of their life's calling. The health care providers are just as frustrated as the patients are.

Instead of assuming everyone is a jerk until proven otherwise, it is just as accurate but more constructive (and compassionate) to assume everyone is lonely and hurting until proven otherwise.

To reach through the cloud of insanity and build a relationship with the doctor: do something silly to grab their attention, hug them, ask them how they're doing, bring them cookies, compliment them, or do whatever you would do in order to get anyone to like you, white lab coat or not.

In other words, act sort of like you are on a date.

• • •

Consider the Source

In eleventh grade we had to write a term paper for history class, and I decided to write about the Ku Klux Klan. I had heard passing mention of the KKK, but I didn't know anything about it. Keep in mind that I was living in South Carolina, a relatively poor state with a very small budget for things like education and books.

I went to the library to research my term paper, and I could only find one book on the topic, which in retrospect was probably KKK recruiting literature. According to this book (my sole source of information for my term paper), the KKK was just a fraternal order, a bunch of guys who liked to hang out and pull pranks on people. They were harmless.

It was quite a while before I learned anything more on the KKK. I don't know what's more disturbing—that the only book I could find on the KKK was their propaganda handbook, or that my teacher gave me an *A*.

Luckily, the KKK was not recruiting in my town, or if they were, they weren't looking for sixteen-year-old girls, so no real harm came of my reading and believing their "innocent" propaganda. But had I been an angry eighteen-year-old boy from a broken family who read and believed that book—in other words, had I been vulnerable on top of gullible—I'd have been ripe pickings for the Klan.

A few years later, I found myself going to various "doc-in-a-box" urgent care centers to treat my symptoms. Finally, I was diagnosed with lupus. What the heck is lupus? Well, since I had no regular doctor, no one took the time to explain the illness to me.

This was before the Internet was widely available to the public. So here I was again at the library, the building that houses both the Bible and propaganda for the KKK, the great philosophers and *Walter the Farting Dog*. The whole world is at your fingertips in the library, but where to begin?

I started with what seemed like an obvious comprehensive source: the encyclopedia. Here's what I learned: do *not* rely on encyclopedias, or any single source, for up-to-date health information. According to the *World Book*, people with systemic lupus died within five years of diagnosis. This time, I *was* vulnerable, and using only one source of information left me believing I had five years to live. I'd never get married, or have kids, or get a master's degree. I wasn't even sure I wanted a master's degree—or kids—but it would be nice to have a choice about it. I was so overwhelmed that I got lost driving home—in my own neighborhood.

There was no mention of hope—such as relief of painful symptoms or regaining my strength and vitality—of any kind. For months I thought I had only a short time to live and nothing to live for. Part of the blame went to the way our medical system works (you can't get any treatment without a specialist, but you might not be able to get in to see a specialist for three to six months) but another part of the problem was using only one information source. Had I had a second source of information, almost *any* second source, I would have known that the information in the encyclopedia was outdated and that, with treatment, I still had a shot at a long life.

Once I finally got some up-to-date information, I wasn't happy with that either. The only solution offered was toxic drugs leading to more illnesses. In this great big universe, there had to be more than one choice, especially when that one choice was so unpalatable. Also, the disease was considered chronic; incurable. I suppose a life sentence is better than a death sentence, but not by much.

I started reading everything I could get my hands on regarding my illness, body-mind connection, alternative medicine, healing diets—one topic leading to another. I called people, I wrote letters, I went to all kinds of alternative practitioners, and I asked lots of questions, even when it wasn't appreciated very much (some doctors just want to hand out orders). This was the term paper of my life. For every one book I read on the problem (my illness), I read twenty or more on solutions: wellness, healing, beating the odds, positive thinking.

Now I believe that I can live for decades, and that if I am willing to make good choices on a daily basis, I can go into complete remission, stay there, and live symptom-free. If I do end up relapsing, I know what to do to get it under control quickly. First choice: tons of acupuncture and qigong (pronounced *chee gong*, it's a gentle healing art much like tai chi, with slow movements and deep breathing). If my organs are failing, then I'll also use immune suppressants to stop the illness. (This is all under the assumption that my life is in balance and my diet is not garbage, of course. If it is, then add "balance life" and "stop eating crap" to the plan.)

I feel empowered by the things I've learned, and I feel I have a great deal of control over how good my health is. When it mattered the most, I finally learned the lesson: consult more than one source.

• • •

You Can't Hide Your Money in an Air Mattress

I thought I had given up my last shred of dignity when I was reduced to wearing puffy slippers and a cheap wig due to my illness. But I still had one shred left, which I surrendered when I finally gave in and filed for bankruptcy. I have since learned that two-thirds of the bankruptcies in this country are caused by medical problems, and I'm not sure that number is high enough to reflect reality.

When I went to my bankruptcy hearing, they asked me a bunch of rapid-fire questions about whether I had any stocks, was married, owned a home, and so on. But they never asked me why I was going bankrupt. Since I paid for all my prescriptions on my credit card, it just looked like I had the classic living-beyond-my-means consumer debt. I was upset that I never got a chance to tell them I didn't spend the money on designer stilettos and a trip to Fiji—I spent it on immune suppressants and a trip to the ER. *Whee.*

Once upon a time, I had a job, savings, and mutual funds and I owned my own small home. I was responsible. After my strokes, I lived in various friends' guest rooms. At one point I was living in a friend's un-air-conditioned computer room, sleeping on an air mattress. Of course, if you're going to live in a spare room, you might as well be broke, too, because you can't hide your money in an air mattress. Even though my dusty boxes of books were in climate-controlled storage, living better than I was, I considered myself fortunate to have family and friends who would take me in. I realized how easily someone could end up broke *and* homeless.

The United States is the only industrialized nation in the world whose government does not provide health care for all of its citizens. We are also, not coincidentally, the only industrialized nation in the world in which two-thirds of the bankruptcies are caused by illness.

You Can Biopsy Me When I'm Dead: My Ten Least-Favorite Medical Procedures

To know what you prefer instead of humbly saying Amen to what the world tells you you ought to prefer is to have kept your soul alive.

—Robert Louis Stevenson

There are travel guides for Europe and Disney filled with can't-miss attractions. Here I present to you, after more research than I really wanted to do, my list of must-miss health care "attractions."

10. *Catheter insertion*

    The hospital staff inserted a catheter, got nothing (no pee), and then wanted to do another one. I said, "I can get enough urinary tract infections on my own without having a tube threaded up into my bladder. Tell your boss 'patient refused procedure.' " Did you know you could refuse procedures? Yup. If they want pee, they'll just have to leave the water running in the sink and show me pictures of Niagara Falls.

9. *Cauterizing (burning!) veins*

Holy crap! How did I get talked into this one? I went to the dermatologist about something else, and he talked me into getting all the little red veins on my nose cauterized. That closes them off for cosmetic reasons, eventually leaving nice, smooth white skin around my nose. It hurt like the dickens and smelled like someone was grilling hamburgers on my face. Then, for the next three weeks, it looked like I had lost a boxing match. My nose was completely purple. The worst part is, I got in an argument with my boyfriend long-distance over the phone, and he sent me a singing telegram to apologize. You should have seen the look on the singer's face, singing an apology song to a girl with a hideously bruised nose.

8. *Iodine test*

I can't believe they don't routinely ask people if they are allergic to iodine before they shoot it into their veins. If you are allergic to shrimp, you should not get an iodine test—it could kill you. And you won't even get the satisfaction of a tasty shrimp cocktail as your last meal.

7. *Hospital roommate getting an enema*

Me, I feel better after a good enema, but I feel much worse after the person in the next bed, who has blockage and hasn't gone to the bathroom in months, has an enema. Geez! And I was in with nausea and stomach flu that time. Private room, anyone?

6. *Getting branded with a permanent marker*

   Okay, if I write on myself with a marker to keep the doctor from lopping off a leg by mistake while I'm knocked out, that's one thing, but when the nurse puts big permanent-marker Xs on my swollen feet where she found my pulse, that's dehumanizing. (Could I at least get a happy face? A flower? Work with me here.)

5. *Kidney biopsy*

   I've had two kidney biopsies. The first time, I told them I was a bleeder—it takes me a long time to clot. There are lots of major vessels in the kidneys, so they cut me open to make sure they didn't hit a major artery and have me bleed to death. They stuck a tube down my throat, cut my side open, and grabbed a piece of tissue. Then the wound got infected. I'm allergic to so many antibiotics that I decided to kill the infection by taking fifty garlic pills a day. Then I sprained my ankle. So there I was, taking ten garlic pills every few hours, hobbling around on crutches in the middle of July, pouring sweat off me, and smelling like a walking plate of pesto. I was safe from vampires at least.

   The end result of all this hassle? The tissue samples were too small to be conclusive, and my drug regimen remained unchanged. When they asked me about doing another kidney biopsy recently, I told them, "You can biopsy me when I'm dead."

4. *EMG (electromyography)*

This should be called OMG! Who the *%^# came up with this test? Especially for someone with nerve damage. Hello?! I'm already in pain! You're zapping me with increasing amounts of voltage, so you can't be surprised when my legs jerk around in reflex. "Stop jerking!" "Stop zapping, and I'll stop jerking." I never got past the first area of testing, my left ankle. Apparently they do both ankles, both knees, hands, elbows, and maybe some other parts. I stood it as long as I could, but I was in so much pain that I didn't even get 20 percent through the test. Apparently, I missed the big finale, where they stick a gigantic needle in your arm and fry the daylights out of you. I never even saw the neurologist. I told my rheumatologist how awful it was, and she said, "Oh, I had one. It wasn't that bad." (Do you have nerve pain? No? Then shut up!)

3. *Blood draw by a bad phlebotomist* (Meaning, they can't find a vein with a needle.)

I swear, some phlebotomists can't find a garden hose with a needle. However, the worst ones are not the actual phlebotomists—the worst are the out-of-practice doctors *playing* phlebotomist. I never let a doctor stick me. I get the expert. If the doctor tries to stick me himself, I say, "Doctor, I think someone's beeping you. Send the phlebotomist, please."

2. *Finger stick* (drawing blood from a fingertip with a spring-loaded needle)

Ow! Do they do this to POWs to get info out of them? I'd squeal in a second! I will never understand why in this age of modern technology they have to pick the one part of my body with the most nerve endings—my fingertips—and slam a spring-loaded needle into it to get a drop of blood. Really, just about anywhere else short of my eyeball would hurt less. How about one of my butt cheeks? Plenty of cushion there.

1. *Bone marrow test*
   Good gravy, this was painful! They put a hole in one side of your back, just above the hip; stick a gigantic needle into your bone, and draw marrow from the inside of your leg. You can feel it all the way to the tip of your big toe. I used up every cuss word I'd ever heard, went through the Fred Flintstone mock swearwords, and then had to make up more. Don't bother to "dress up" for this test. Okay, I admit I had a crush on my hematologist, so I wore some cute, flowery Victoria's Secret undies to my bone marrow test. What a waste! Blood gets all over them.

Learn about a test before you agree to submit to one. I realize sometimes they are necessary, but beware of doctors who are "test happy," and remember that you have the right to say no. It's not their body, and they are not the ones who live with the long- or short-term ramifications of these decisions. Or the bills. Or the ruined Victoria's Secret lingerie.

● ● ●

Send In the Clowns!

A clown is like an aspirin, only he works twice as fast.
—Groucho Marx

Once upon a time, there were no rock stars. There were only church musicians, who humbly served the congregation with no applause, and court musicians, who served at the pleasure of the royals. Musicians were basically servants.

Then along came Beethoven, who demanded that he be catered to and listened to, and who was positively outraged if anyone dared to have a conversation while he was performing. The musician went from serving the public to demanding that they worship him, and the rock star was born.

This attitude has spread to some pretty weird places, such as reality TV competitions for everything from dancing and cooking to grooming dogs and cutting hair. Every single one of these shows features people who are good at what they do and therefore think they should be treated like rock stars. But really, how much more humble of a profession is there than cooking?

Or, for heaven's sake, trimming a dog's toenails? We've forgotten that we are put on earth to serve each other, from the janitor to the teacher to, yes, the CEO. Jesus himself washed his disciples' feet, so if you truly had a "god complex," you would be serving others at every opportunity.

Before the twentieth century, doctors learned medicine by apprenticeship. It was a humble profession, and they were basically indentured servants. I don't know who is responsible for the change that turned doctors into rock stars, but somehow it's been forgotten that doctors serve patients, not the other way around. I suspect this can be largely blamed on their education (or should I say hazing) in medical school, which was described by Dean Wilcott in the movie *Patch Adams* (based on a true story) this way:

"Our job is to rigorously and ruthlessly train the humanity out of you and make you into something better. We're gonna make doctors out of you."

Better than a human being? That means the schools are either trying to make doctors into robots that don't make mistakes or gods who know everything. Or worse, a rock star. Either way, I don't want a doctor who has lost her humanity.

Voltaire said, "The art of medicine consists of keeping the patient amused while nature heals the disease." If you're a doctor using this approach, that kind of makes you like a clown. (A clown who dresses really blah.) Patch Adams, MD, understands this, and that's why he's famous for wearing a red rubber nose and "clowning around" with his patients.

When a clown comes into the room, it's not about him—it's about you. The clown knows he is there to serve his fellow man—to amuse, to distract, and to bring good cheer. He doesn't care how big a fool he makes of himself, as long as you laugh. In fact, his job is to make a fool of himself. And though I'm sure it's only a matter of time before we have a reality show pitting clowns against one another to see who's the best (and who deserves rock star status, a million bucks, and a TV show), for now most clowns know their job is a humble (though honorable and vital) profession.

When a rock star comes into a room, it's all about her and her ego. We're supposed to feel lucky just to have her breeze by on her way to her next Important Thing to Do. When I'm afraid and in pain, I don't want to be cared for by a rock star. At that moment, I really need someone to care about me. Forget the rock star. Send in the clowns!

• • •

Death Is Not Psychosomatic

For some reason, doctors don't seem to like to diagnose people with autoimmune diseases. It is common for someone with an autoimmune disease to suffer and go to several different doctors over the course of several years before finally getting a diagnosis. We're constantly being told it's nothing, or it's psychosomatic (caused entirely by our emotions, all in our heads). I didn't realize kidney failure, anemia, stroke, congestive heart failure, neuropathy, edema, and migraines were all psychosomatic. What irony, then, that there is no psychologist available at the hospital. Still, I'm pretty sure that at least death is not psychosomatic, and that thousands of people die from autoimmune diseases every year.

Even if I *could* conjure up an illness at will, being sick is a lot of bother to go to in order to get five minutes of a doctor's time. There are far more efficient ways to get attention. For example: streaking, getting a mohawk, running for public office, and screaming about how sick people get too much attention. If I could pick, I'd choose any of those over having an autoimmune disease. Because, unlike having a chronic illness, you can stop doing those things anytime you want.

• • •

My Other Body Is a Porsche

Some patients I see are actually draining into their bodies the diseased thoughts of their minds.

—Zachary T. Bercvoitz, MD

I've heard numerous doctors compare the human body to an automobile: you have to do regular maintenance, give it good fuel, etc. There's even a book called *You: The Owner's Manual*. It's a pretty good analogy, to a point, but it has a few shortcomings.

First of all, there are a couple of things we have that a car doesn't (and I don't mean anatomically): a mind and a soul. Without a driver (mind), the car doesn't go anywhere, and unlike most humans, a car can function just fine with no soul (insert joke about your boss here).

Whether we like it or not, human beings are higher maintenance than your typical car. We all know that if your body is in bad shape, everything else in your life is going to suffer, but we have emotional needs and mental health that also require regular attention. If you are sad, lonely, and filled with unhealthy thoughts, all the vitamins and health food in the world are not going to heal you. We are a three-part being (mind, body, soul), and each of the three parts has to be in working condition for the other two to function properly.

Another limitation of the car-as-human analogy is that you can't trade in your body for a new one. I asked. During the stroke/kidney failure/congestive heart failure/anemia/edema/neuropathy episode, I felt like I had gotten stuck with one of those old, finicky, run-down, noisy, smoke-spewing eyesore Porsches that people swear they're going to fix up one day. Only in my case, it wasn't a spare car cluttering up the garage—it was my only vehicle.

I was so disgusted with all the crazy, seemingly random stuff my body was doing and the constant pain and exhaustion, I asked my doctor if I could get a full-body transplant. Apparently, this is not an option. (I do hear, however, that you can swap in your soul for a gold fiddle.)

My point here—and I do have one—is that if we're going to use the car analogy, then let's make sure to put a driver in the seat and talk about her care and feeding, too. A race car does not win the Indy 500 by itself. I'm not just a machine; I am a person. I'm not asking that doctors provide all the love, comfort, prayer, humor, and optimism that I need to nourish my soul. I'm merely asking that they acknowledge its existence, and perhaps open their minds to the fact that the state of the soul affects the state of the body. My illness is not "all in my head," but my health is likewise not all "in my body."

• • •

Thanks for Not Accidentally Killing Me

I noticed as I was reading through my own hospital records that my father had died of stomach cancer. As he is very much alive, I'm sure both he and his stomach would be surprised to hear this. Fortunately, that was a harmless error, but at this point I've had so many different tests and pills and doctors that I consider myself fortunate that I'm not maimed or dead from a hospital mistake.

In 1995 the *Journal of the American Medical Association* reported that 280,000 patients die every year from hospital-related injuries in this country. (If this is the number given by an industry reporting on itself, you can probably guess that this estimate is low.) There are also upward of 3,000 "wrong-site" operations a year. That means they operated on the wrong part of the body—or on the wrong patient! While things go right most of the time, that's not good enough for someone who's just had his one good foot removed.

Want to steer clear of that kind of fun? Here are a few ideas to help you avoid "death by health care":

- Idiot-proof yourself before you go under. If you're being operated on, write on yourself with a permanent marker. Write your name and why you are being operated on ("gall bladder," "right hip," etc.).

- Advertise your allergies. If you are allergic to iodine, or latex, or anything that might make you go anaphylactic (swell up and stop breathing), write it everywhere. Not just on your chart, because—sorry to say—in my experience not many people look at it. Don't just tell one nurse, because nurses change shifts. Don't just tell the doctor, because doctors see a zillion patients and spend the rest of their time fending off drug reps and fighting with insurance companies. *You* have to remember, and if you're asleep or doped up, you can't stop them.

  Ideally, you would have a patient advocate—a private nurse, a friend or a relative, or a professional—there at all times. But that's usually not the case, so put big signs up above your headboard and on the door, use stickers on the front of your chart clipboard or on your food tray, or write on your arms IODINE ALLERGY! LATEX ALLERGY (unless you have an ink allergy). If you have a latex allergy and end up in the hospital, have them remove the box of latex gloves from the room and bring in nonlatex gloves. If you're about to get a needle, ask before they wipe with a swab whether they're using iodine.

- Ask questions. For example, if doctors want to send you for a test where you're about to get injected with a dye, ask what the dye is, in case you're allergic. In the case of an iodine test, someone who is allergic to shrimp will not be able to tolerate iodine, and this can result in death. This is entirely preventable, but doctors don't routinely ask people beforehand. All they have to say is, "Are you allergic to shrimp?" If you are, then you're allergic to iodine. Why can't this be a law? They've certainly managed to institute mandatory questioning before X-rays:

"Are you pregnant?"

"Lord, no!" (The last thing I want to do when I'm in chronic pain is have sex. Not that I'm getting a lot of offers anyway when I'm lying around miserable and unkempt.)

"When was your last period?"

"Oh, months ago. I have no idea." (Mine stops when I'm sick.)

"Are you sure you're not pregnant?"

"Not unless it was immaculate conception."

Now they're confused, and we start all over again.

If only they would grill people as rigorously about allergies. It would take five seconds to ask a question that could save someone's life, and it wouldn't be nearly as embarrassing!

- Remind the doctors of their oath. I think in addition to announcing my allergies on big neon signs on my chart and hospital door, I'll write on my forehead: FIRST DO NO HARM.

• • •

A Good Vein Is Hard to Find: Two Sticks and You're Out!

It doesn't matter how many times I get my blood taken, or an IV put in, or chelation or chemo—I never get used to it. I have this theory that a little controlled bloodletting may actually be good for me, however. So when I get my blood taken, I think, "Here's a chance for my body to make some fresh new blood!" It doesn't make the needle hurt any less, but it does make me feel better about having to go through it.

However, I hit my limit when the resident who was overseeing my case in the hospital tried—and failed—to insert an IV needle into my arms four times. I finally put both arms behind my back where she couldn't get to them and said, "You need to give up." She said—with great melodrama—"Oh Carla, I'll never give up on you."

Once I stopped laughing, I said, "No, not on me. You need to give up on *you* ever getting a vein on my arm. Send me a pediatric nurse!" Kids have small veins, so pediatric nurses are good with folks whose veins are hard to find, and they use "baby needles," which are smaller, easier to use, and hurt less.

The rule among the nurses is: two sticks and you're out. Apparently, nurses get performance anxiety, too, and once they fail twice to get a vein, they are to pass the task to someone else. Doctors don't seem to be in on this little rule, which is unfortunate, because in my experience they are the absolute *worst* at using needles. Doctors don't do it every day, so they're rusty (rusty skills and needles do not go well together!). If they're not going to enforce the two sticks rule on themselves, I will.

• • •

A Hundred Dollars for Your Thoughts

I resisted the idea of going to a therapist because I thought, "Why should I have to pay someone to listen to me? Isn't that what friends are for?" Well, in an ideal world, yes, but we do not live in an ideal world. In fact, we live in a culture with a severe deficiency in people who are willing and able to listen to one another. I mean really listen—without interrupting, without mentally wandering off somewhere else, without judging, without quick-fixing.

When I first fell ill, there were so many emotions to deal with, it was just too much for the average friend to take in. It's even harder for family members, who often have their own batch of powerful emotions regarding your illness. Plus, they're not always sure which things you mention are confidential and which are lunch-table fodder.

So I decided to hire someone to yell at for an hour a week. Someone who didn't know any of my friends and therefore couldn't break confidence, even if she wanted to, and someone who couldn't take my problems and somehow turn them around and make it about herself. I needed some therapy.

Of course, not all therapists are created equal. For starters, the big difference between psychologists and psychiatrists is that a psychiatrist can prescribe medication. A psychologist cannot, so the psychologist *has* to listen to you! He can't just get out a prescription pad and put you out of *his* misery. I went to a psychologist.

It was such a relief to be able to speak my truth to another person without interruption or drama. I vented and vented, and every single week before I left I stopped by the bathroom to take a humongous dump. What a beautiful metaphor.

I only went to that therapist six times, because during the last visit she told me I needed to accept my illness and stop running around looking for alternative therapies. You might say I dumped her. Up to that point she hadn't really given any advice, so things were going fine. I think I got the message that she was tired of listening to my venting, and that was okay—I was just about done anyway. I had hired her so I could yell, and I was done yelling. It was time to move on to the next thing.

Psychologists are a wonderful help, but they can't replace real friends. It's kind of a one-sided relationship where the patient does all the talking. You never really know much about psychologists. You can't call them at home, you don't know where they live, and if you fall off the face of the earth, they may never find out. On the other hand, friends don't always keep things confidential, and they are not always able to listen without interrupting, getting distracted, or trying to fix things.

When you're in a lot of pain, you sometimes find yourself with a choice between friends who care but don't know how to listen and psychologists who know how to listen but, as a matter of survival, don't really care that deeply. So, I was understandably excited when I discovered a caring community of great listeners in Re-evaluation Counseling (RC, aka co-counseling). The Re-evaluation Counseling organization advocates peer counseling— that is, people counsel each other mostly by active listening (listening intently while saying very little and allowing the speaker to work through his or her own problems). Counselors take turns, first counseling, then being counseled. With the exception of special optional weekend workshops, no money changes hands. The goal, as with any counseling, is to break out of old destructive patterns and to think clearly. To find people doing RC near you, check out www.rc.org. If you can't find an RC group, join an online support group or start your own in a community center like I did—just four of us, meeting once a month, sharing both concerns and things that were helping us. And nobody pays anybody else to listen.

• • •

Teaching People How to Treat You

Have you ever left a doctor's office wondering how in the world the office was still in business? If you must go to a doctor—and if you've got a chronic illness, you must—save yourself some frustration and ask friends, family, and trusted doctors for a referral first. Now that I've figured out the referral process, I will never go back to my old system of just grabbing some name out of the phone book. Of course, sometimes you've got no choice. Or rather, a choice of one.

The two years I was on Medicaid, I had extremely limited choices in care, and I had to go to a lot of "ologists": nephrologist, hematologist, rheumatologist. In addition, I was going to an osteopath for chelation therapy, and an acupuncturist. My life was an endless stream of appointments, and I frequently had more than one appointment a day. There was only one hematologist, one rheumatologist, one psychiatrist, and one nephrologist in the county who would accept Medicaid (it doesn't pay much).

I needed them, but they didn't need me, so they had me over a barrel: I just had to put up with their limited hours and rude office staff. Particularly at the hematologist's office.

At this office, two hours past my actual appointment time was the normal wait. Then I would get my blood taken and wait another thirty to forty minutes in the back. It made me mad that I had to be on time, but they had complete disregard for my time. When I teach guitar lessons, if I'm not there when the lesson is supposed to start, or I'm running fifteen minutes behind schedule, the student leaves and I don't get paid.

Maybe it wouldn't be so aggravating if once I finally saw the doctor he spent more than two minutes with me, or if there was some explanation or an apology—or if it didn't happen every single time (I was at that office two to four times a month). It was clear they were just booking too many people, like airlines that sell more seats than they actually have, assuming someone won't show up.

Still, I figured I had no choice in the matter—I was severely anemic, they were the only game in town, and they knew it. So I started bringing a picnic lunch and my notebook of song ideas to make better use of the time. If I was at home, that's what I would be doing anyway—writing or having a snack. This was working so well that I was actually disappointed when it was time for me to go in—"hang on a sec, I think I've finally fixed the chorus of this song!"

Then one day I had an appointment at the hematologist at 1:00 p.m. and the acupuncturist at 4:00 p.m.— and the acupuncturist runs on time. It was getting past 3:00 p.m., they had brought me to the back but I still hadn't seen the doctor, and I needed time to drive to the other appointment. So I got up and left.

I didn't yell or make a scene. That's the difference between being assertive and being aggressive—I simply set a boundary and matter-of-factly told the receptionist I had another appointment and couldn't wait any longer. The next time I was there, I was seen a lot faster, and when the doctor saw me waiting in the exam room, he said, "I'll be right there. Don't leave." I gently but clearly taught them that day what I was willing to tolerate.

Then there are people who just can't be taught how to treat anyone. At one point, my general practitioner sent me to a psychiatrist, because I was having a hard time coping with the mood swings caused by the prednisone. So I went there thinking, "Great! Finally, someone to talk to for an hour, to help me sort out my problems."

Well, this psychiatrist was also seeing all Medicaid patients. She made all appointments for 10:00 a.m. (about a dozen of us were in the waiting room with the same appointment time), and then she showed up about an hour later.

When she asked me, "How are you doing?" I assumed she actually wanted to know how I was doing. Turns out it was more of a New York City "How ya doin'," which is supposed to be responded to with another "How ya doin'," neither of which is supposed to be answered with how anyone is actually doing. I realized this when she held up her hand while I was in midsentence and said, "I don't have time to listen to your problems. Your Medicaid does not pay that much." She spent about one to two minutes with each of us, just enough time to write a prescription.

If you think something is wrong with this picture, you're right. Two years later, she was arrested for Medicaid fraud. For each one-minute visit with a patient, she was billing Medicaid for an hour. I, in the meantime, had just written her off and stopped going after two visits (why I even went a second time I can't say).

While I believe that anyone can change, the person has to want to change. At that point, the psychiatrist was quite happy with how things were (at least until the arrest). Sometimes the relationship just can't be fixed. All you can do is love yourself enough to leave and move on to someone who interacts with you appropriately. And who knows, maybe that psychiatrist will eventually learn something about how to treat people. I'm sure there are lots of "teachable moments" in jail.

"Sittin' in the Waiting Room"

(Sing to the tune of "Personality")

I'm at the gynecologist (whoops!)

Phlebotomist (stab!)

Proctologist (hey!)

Psychologist (hmm . . .)

Urologist I waited for two hours and

Then I saw him walking to his car

Office hours were over—they were over!

I knew what I had to do

I ran him over and over

Left him in the waiting room

• • •

Post-partial Depression

I found something I hate more than getting a pap smear: going to the dentist, mostly because of how much the Novocain shot hurts. One time when I went to the dentist, I actually had to get two shots, because I could still feel the drill after the first one. But the drill didn't really hurt, so I asked the dentist not to give me a second shot, but she did anyway. The second that Novocain entered my system I instantly felt like crying.

Puzzled by my reaction, I gathered enough of my senses to look it up online several days later. Once I finally figured out how to spell Novocain, it all fell into place. (FYI, the generic version has an *e* at the end, and if you search online using this spelling, you will find a song by Green Day and a weird movie of the same name.)

According to Drugs.com, the Food and Drug Administration advises using as low a dosage as possible to avoid adverse side effects, and it warns against using Novocain on patients with known drug allergies, of which I have several. (Several drugs give me a full-body rash, one makes my tongue swell up, one makes me hurl, and latex makes my skin feel like it's burning. Now I can add another drug reaction to my repertoire: "instant psycho.")

So with several drug allergies listed on my chart, why did I get not one, but two shots? I ended up with a six-day attack of fibromyalgia, of which I had been free for several months; severe anxiety; and major mood swings. Plus a bill for $750. Oh, but they validated my parking, and I got some free floss. I recovered, but only after two weeks of lengthy back-to-back acupuncture treatments. If I did not have a fantastic and available acupuncturist, I would still be suffering instead of sitting here typing about this in the past tense.

The main lessons I want to share from this experience are these:

First, if you have any drug sensitivities, you may not want to use Novocain. I have learned, via my pointing and clicking, that there is a far more hypoallergenic drug available—Lidocaine—that will provide the same numbing. In the future, I will list Novocain (and novocaine) as a drug allergy so that I do not have to go through this again. Hey, Lidocaine may not work for you, but the point is, ask questions and learn about alternatives.

Second, before embarking on major dental procedures, make sure your health is stable enough to handle the procedure and you have some form of support (such as acupuncture or another form of complementary care) to help you get back to yourself afterward.

Third, before making an appointment, decide whether you want a mercury-free dentist. Mercury is a toxic element, yet some dentists still use fillings that contain this element. Those fillings are called amalgams, and they are silver in color. I prefer fillings that are completely gold, platinum, or composite. I also pass on the fluoride.

Finally, a dentist, just like a doctor, is definitely someone you should get a recommendation for. I do that when I'm looking for a hairdresser or a mechanic, and they don't even affect my health. Of all people, shouldn't a dentist be found by word of *mouth?*

• • •

Doctors Are People, Too

This may come as a shock to some of you, but I recently learned that doctors are people. Not only that, but when they leave their office, they think about us and dream about us. As much as medical school tries to beat it out of them, they are still human beings. Not only do they affect us, we—the patients—affect them.

Many folks have put doctors up on a pedestal and never question anything they do or say, which is how you can end up getting lots of unnecessary tests and procedures. Such patients have an unhealthy respect for authority. While these are "easy" patients for the doctor to deal with, they are passive, and that is not the profile of a survivor.

I, however, have a sometimes unhealthy disrespect for authority. I approach authority figures with a chip on my shoulder and an assumption that they are going to harm me, through either self-interest or negligence. I'm a royal pain, a "problem" patient who comes in with challenging questions and a batch of her own ideas about how things should be done. What's good about this is that I'm participating in my own recovery, which sends very positive messages to my mind and body about my hope and belief in my survival. What's bad about it is that it makes it difficult to form a trusting relationship when I always assume anyone in authority is an incompetent idiot until proven otherwise.

Though some doctors have a demeanor resembling something between a robot and a block of ice, underneath that is a person with—gasp!—feelings and insecurities, and hostility is only going to put more walls between us. But I'm still not putting my life in the hands of someone who's only known me for a few minutes.

Somewhere between too deferential and too hostile is probably a healthy approach that involves mutual respect and a spirit of cooperation, a team effort where both parties participate in the decisions and each is a little vulnerable.

This really hit home for me at the nephrologist one day. After his courteous, "How are you doing?" and I said, "Okay; how are you?" he teared up as he told me how much stress he was under. He only accepted Medicaid patients—the neediest, sickest of patients, with the lowest insurance reimbursement—and had patients with AIDS and who were in and out of emergency rooms. Then he had the insurance company calling him and grilling him about every single test he ordered.

I asked him why he took only Medicaid patients, and he told me he felt he needed to give back because his entire education had been paid for with grants and scholarships. Every visit after that, he would tell me his troubles. I don't think anyone else in his life ever took the time to ask him how *he* was doing.

Now granted, his crying in front of me every time I came in made me a little uncomfortable, but I'm glad it happened, because it helped me see doctors for what they are: regular people under a lot of stress. I no longer saw him as an authority figure. He became a real person to me, someone I cared about.

• • •

A Picture Is Worth a Thousand Doctor Appointments

Based on the radical notion that maybe doctors are human beings, I wondered how far this idea might go. Might they be impressionable, just like we mere mortals? Is it possible that if they've only ever seen me pale and weak, they have trouble imagining me any other way?

I had numerous specialists, and I wanted them to be in agreement with me about a good outcome, so I gave them each a picture of me onstage when I was healthy and asked them to put it at the front of my medical chart. I wanted them to see the healthy me, a vibrant, smiling young woman playing the guitar with ease. In my mind, that is the real me, and I needed them to catch a glimpse of it. Not to be used as "look at what I've lost" but as "here's where we're going," like a map.

All any of them had ever seen was a pale, anemic weakling with a cane and compression stockings. I got a few of them on board with me, to at least consider the possibility that I could again be vibrant and energetic. Maybe even completely well. I wanted them to treat me like someone who had a promising future.

My osteopath took to calling me his "miracle child" because he saw me the most, and every week under his care I got better and stronger. The more he believed in me, the more encouraged I was, and the harder I worked at getting better. With his enthusiasm, he taught me that I could have a caring, nonadversarial relationship with a doctor, and both of us got something out of it: I got healthier, and his work was validated.

Now that I've recovered my looks, my health, and my guitar-playing skills, the next thing on my to-do list is to get back in touch with all the various doctors who have seen me in my worst state, to let them know I got better. It seems like no one ever does this, so doctors only see sick people. Eventually this has to wear on them and make them believe on some level that no one ever really gets better, which causes them to make absolute statements (like the one who told me, "You'll be on dialysis within five years") without leaving any room for hope.

If people like me, who regain all their kidney function without a transplant, were to get back in touch with these folks and say, "Hey! I got better!" it might make the doctors' day a little brighter, who, in turn, might make all their patients' day a little brighter. Even more important, maybe they would leave a little wiggle room for hope when they hand out the next prognosis. Instead of an absolute "Dialysis within five years," the doctor now might say, "Most folks in your situation end up on dialysis. But some get better."

• • •

This Is (Not) Your Life

When my first major health fiasco hit, I was twenty-five and working full-time in a retail musical instrument store, and I had health insurance. The illness cost me both the job and the insurance, among other things, and left with me a pre-existing condition, which made it impossible to obtain new medical insurance. Because of this, when my second major health fiasco happened, I had no insurance, so I went to a teaching hospital where they took indigent patients. (*Indigent* means no money, not to be confused with *indigenous*, which means "native people," such as Aborigines or Native Americans. Although I was born in a hospital, so I guess I was indigenous as well as indigent.)

After I was sprung from the joint, my follow-up appointments with the kidney doctor were set at the indigent clinic. Well, the clinic sees all its patients on either Tuesday or Thursday. I was a Tuesday patient, and all of us had the same appointment time: 9:00 a.m. It was first-come, first served, so we all showed up at 7:30 a.m. At 9:00 they would start calling us to get our weight and blood pressure, and then we were herded back to the waiting room to wait some more, usually until about noon. All of us had kidney failure, so we sat there with the water draining down to our ankles, our legs swelling bigger by the hour. Sometime around noon (three ankle inches and a half a box of Cheez-Its later), I would get my few minutes with the doctor.

The final insult was that I had a different doctor every time I went. That meant I had to give my entire medical history and relive all the bleak, dark, traumatic crap I was trying so hard to not think about, like a really depressing episode of *This Is Your Life*. About the third time, I had had enough. I brought in a typed, thirteen-page medical history with all my illnesses, allergies, symptoms, surgeries, corresponding dates, and the names and addresses of all the doctors I could remember. I handed it to the new doc, and he said, "Oh, no. I have to take your history orally." Instead of suggesting another orifice where he could "take it," I restrained myself and I said, "Why? So you can pretend to have a rapport with me?"

I mean, it's not like he was going to be there next month, and it's not like the next doc was going to be able to read anything he wrote on my chart. Furthermore, when you're on nine drugs, your memory is not exactly tack-sharp. But I guess this was more about him learning to take a patient history than it was about how it affected my mental health to keep going through this process over and over. After all, it was a teaching hospital.

While my Mr. One-Night Stand of a doctor wasn't interested in my hours of meticulous record compilation, I did create a valuable resource that other folks do find useful, especially alternative practitioners such as acupuncturists. A lot of us with chronic illnesses do keep a health file of our own, because if you move to another town or go to several specialists, or ever need to file for disability, you really have to be the keeper of your own file. (For details about what kind of information to include in your personal health file, see the "Patient, Heal Thyself" essay.)

Doctors (even those who actually do have a rapport with you) routinely throw records away after seven years, and then they are *gone*. If you don't have your own copies, pull up a chair and prepare for an encore presentation of *This Is Your Life*. It seems to me that the more times you repeat something, the further it becomes engrained in your consciousness, kind of like when my mom made me memorize our address and phone number when I was in first grade. Every morning before I walked to school, my mom made me recite it. Even though we lived at this address for only a year and I was just six years old, to this day I remember it, in the sing-songy way I used to play it back to Mom: *390 Thirty-second Street, 654–4233.*

While that's a fond memory, I have no desire to have a sing-songy list of every health problem I've ever experienced rattling around in my consciousness like a never-ending nightmare. This is the real reason I made my health file, so that I can write it down, get it out of my brain, and think about something else. Like 390 Thirty-second Street. Because this is just my health file. This is not my life.

• • •

Prednisone: Can't Live with It, Can't Live without It

The bad news: you're very, very sick.

    The good news: there is something that can help you.

The bad news: it's prednisone.

    The good news: it's cheap.

The bad news: it causes mood swings.

    The good news: now you have an excuse.

The bad news: it has a lot of other side effects, such as weight gain, moon face, osteoporosis, hair loss, hair growth, cataracts, diabetes, high blood pressure, and insomnia.

    The good news: your kitchen floor will be spotless, your CD collection will be in perfect alphabetical order, and you'll catch up on all those reruns of *Matlock*.

Swap out one disease, get four more, and look and feel like crap in the process. All for only $4 a month at Walmart! What a deal!

I've been on this stuff three times now, for about a year each time. I take it because it works; I complain about it because it is no fun being on it. It's kind of like living with your parents when you're a teenager: you're dependent on them, but they drive you crazy, and hopefully at some point you won't need to live there anymore.

I've always managed to get completely off the prednisone within a year of starting it, using alternative medicine, and sometimes with the help of other, less-toxic medications. When the time comes to get off the prednisone, taper off it slowly, because if you suddenly stop taking it, you can die. (Or worse, you'll end up on an even higher dose of prednisone than you were taking before.) Prednisone replaces cortisol, the hormone that runs your vital organs, and there is a lag time between when you stop taking it and when your body starts making that vital hormone again. I mention this because, yes, we're all supposed to do this under a doctor's supervision, but I know in reality some of us get fed up and decide to just stop taking it. Please, don't suddenly stop. Your body can't recover from that.

I hate prednisone a lot, but I love me more. To immortalize my love-hate (hate-hate?) relationship with this dreaded med, I wrote this little ditty. I borrowed the tune from "Comet (will make your mouth turn green)," an old babysitter classic (the original tune being "Colonel Bogey's March").

"Prednisone"

Prednisone will make you get real fat

Prednisone will give you cataracts

Prednisone it will destroy your bones

So take some prednisone destroy your bones today

Prednisone your moods are up and down

Prednisone your face is big and round

Prednisone will mess with your hormones

So take some prednisone spend your life alone today

Give it to your cat give it to your dog

Give it to your guinea pig

See 'em acting weird see 'em eat a lot see 'em getting really big

Take it for your gout or if you've got a bout

Of poison oak or poison ivy

Take it in a drop, take it in a pill

Take it intravenously

Prednisone you start with one complaint

Prednisone now you've got seven or eight

Prednisone you could be dead you know

So take your prednisone or pick your tombstone today

. . .

Pick Your Poison

I find the medicine worse than the malady.
—John Fletcher, *Love's Cure*, Act 3, Scene 2

Comedian Bernie Mac, dead at fifty. The papers say it was pneumonia. My husband said, "Who dies of pneumonia anymore, especially at age fifty?"

Someone who is on immune-system suppressants, that's who. Bernie Mac had sarcoidosis, an autoimmune disease, and it was being controlled by immune suppressants. The doctors declared his condition to be "in remission," but that remission came at the price of his not being able to fight off pneumonia.

This is frightening for those of us who have been given the choice between dying of kidney failure or having our immune systems squashed, leaving us vulnerable to death by pneumonia and other illnesses that usually would not be life-threatening.

What are we supposed to do? My doctors told me repeatedly that I would not survive if I kept refusing the prednisone. But I resisted taking it for months because I read about all the side effects, which sounded worse than just being in pain. In retrospect,

I think there would be something wrong with me if I *didn't* find the idea of taking prednisone objectionable! Who wants to be a twenty-five-year-old fat, moody, moon-faced, blind, brittle-boned diabetic with no immune system if there is any other possible way to deal with the situation? I was *single*. Can't you just see that match.com ad? Bloated, anemic, moody, bald, pale female seeks—anyone. *Anyone!* Oh, yeah, do I want to date *her*? She sounds so incredibly *needy*.

Your typical hard-core health nut would say, "It's simple. Visit a naturopath, get off all the medications, eliminate junk food, detox, and eat superfoods." This is a fine idea, in principle, and it probably even works—if you have tons of support—as in a staff preparing your foods and providing other therapies.

But anyone who thinks it's "simple" and "obvious" has never had to deal firsthand with either sarcoidosis or any other life-threatening, debilitating chronic illness. I decided to try the naturopathic approach myself the first time I was ill, and let me tell you—when the disease is in attack mode, unless you have someone making your food for you and coming to your house to treat you, you won't have the energy to do the amount of work it takes to get better using naturopathy alone. There is a lot of shopping for fresh food, driving to appointments, preparing the food, and cleaning up. And when I was in the condition I was in at that point, I had to spend a half hour just working up the gumption to get off the sofa to go to the bathroom.

As much as I detest being on drugs, I've found them to be a necessary evil for periods of time in my life. I go on the drugs to stop the disease from destroying my kidneys, lungs, heart, brain, and whatever else it may be attacking. As soon as I start feeling a bit better, I seek out alternative medicine and start doing the things I know I should be doing: acupuncture, gentle exercise, eating less garbage and more real food, doing things I love, and being with people who make me happy. And reading plenty of comic books.

The two approaches work together, and I taper off the drugs as my test results improve. I desperately want to be drug-free, but I more desperately want to have all my original vital organs intact. Point being, it's your life. If I don't want to take prednisone or any other drug, I don't have to, and you don't have to either. They can't make us. If we were children, the government could probably force our parents to give it to us. However, we have to live with the consequences of our decisions, and for me, sometimes taking prednisone for nine months or so is better than being in chronic pain while autoimmune disease eats away at my kidneys.

Taking medication is not a permanent solution; it's just a life raft. Staying on any drug long-term is going to cause as many problems as it solves. Part of the reason I was on prednisone was to save my kidneys, but one of the long-term risks of prednisone is kidney failure! It's not just prednisone; chemotherapy actually increases your risk of getting cancer. Diuretics and aspirin can cause gout. We can't just pop pills, go on with our lives, and expect no consequences.

In my little support group of four people, I saw a few possible futures: one was in a wheelchair, constantly getting surgeries because of the bone thinning caused by medication; another was a hundred pounds overweight because of medication; the third was on and off medication but relapsed every eighteen months. I went searching for alternatives.

The books out there that promise actual healing from autoimmune diseases (as opposed to just coping with them) emphasize three things: taking care of emotional baggage, detoxification, and eating real food (and not eating junk food). If you are willing to work at it, you can reduce or even completely wean off your medications. You should, of course, be monitored with regular blood tests by a physician. (I, regrettably, skipped a few years.) Then maybe, unlike me, you can have just one major health fiasco instead of three.

• • •

Chapter 3

That's Inflammatory! What Not to Eat If You Have an Autoimmune Disease

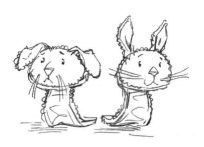

Part 1: What If I Really Am What I Eat?

Let food be your medicine.
—Hippocrates

When you have a chronic illness, it can feel like you're being randomly attacked by some mysterious force.

Scientists have tried to find a genetic cause for autoimmune diseases, without much success. Given that autoimmune diseases are far more common in industrialized nations and have tripled in rate in the last few decades, it's far more likely that diet and environmental pollutants are to blame. President George H. W. Bush and his dog Millie both had autoimmune diseases—that makes a case for environment over genetics. There is one thing more than any other that we have control over: what we eat.

I was pondering all this while munching on a bag of Cheesy Puffs, and I looked at the ingredients list: partially hydrogenated soybean oil, disodium phosphate, artificial flavor, monosodium glutamate, lactic acid, and artificial colors.

Then it struck me: I thought I was a vegetarian, but I'm not! I'm a crapatarian. Just because that Cheesy Puff is made without meat doesn't mean it's healthy. Cyanide doesn't have any meat in it, either. Maybe being vegetarian actually involves eating *vegetables*. I'm not saying my illness was caused entirely by my eating habits, but when your day starts with a diet soda and ends with a candy bar, you shouldn't be too surprised when something goes awry. And I can't get too angry with the doctor for putting chemicals into my body if I'm downing the pills with Nutrasweet and yellow dye #6.

The first time a doctor (an osteopath) discussed diet with me in regards to quelling my autoimmune conditions, I thought, "That's ridiculous. How can what I eat have anything to do with my health?" What's more ridiculous, in retrospect, is thinking that what I eat won't affect me.

What passes for nutritional information in the mainstream media is extremely confusing and contradictory. One week, margarine is a health food. The next week, it's death on a plate.

In the end, all you need are a few simple rules. Eliminate artificial sweeteners and MSG. If you've got an autoimmune condition, try eliminating gluten. Everyone should "Eat food. Not too much. Mostly plants," according to Michael Pollan, author of *In Defense of Food*. Sounds obvious, but a lot of what we chew and swallow is not food; it's not nutritious and can even be harmful. Here's another point to remember courtesy of Joel Fuhrman, author of *Eat to Live*: "The salad is the main course." (Salad means leafy greens.)

Food is not the only trigger for illness, of course. I can't control the fact that planes fly over my house and pollute the air, or that corporations dump poisons in our water, or that I may have a genetic tendency towards autoimmunity. But I *can* control what I put in my mouth.

• • •

Part 2: Getting the Soda Monkey off My Back

If I were to only change one thing about my diet, this is it: eliminate excitotoxins. What is an excitotoxin? The most common culprits are MSG and aspartame (aka NutraSweet, Equal, and AminoSweet). Siegfried Schmidt, MD, claims to have completely cured numerous patients of fibromyalgia simply by eliminating excitotoxins from their diets.

After being warned repeatedly by various health practitioners about the dangers of aspartame, I have finally ended my decades-long romance with diet sodas. I tell you, it's like quitting heroin—without the glamour. I honestly can't recall how many times I tried to quit drinking diet soda before I finally succeeded, and I still fear I'll fall off the wagon. So every time I look at a cold, dripping, tempting bottle of diet something, I tell myself "poison."

There are all kinds of accusations flying around about aspartame. Some say it turns into formaldehyde when it gets into your body. Some say it turns into formaldehyde *before* it enters the body, if the temperature is warm enough (99°F). Aspartame has been implicated in causing kidney problems, cancer, lupus, fibromyalgia, MS, birth defects, tumors, seizures, Gulf War Syndrome, and (ironically) weight gain, among other problems. Yikes! It may be tasty, but nothing is *that* tasty. If these links are real, then this "food" has no place in our diets, in our fridges, in our stores, or in our food chain.

How many of the accusations are true, I'm not sure, although there are an astounding number of studies out on aspartame. (Google it!) But I do know this: there are very few casual diet soda drinkers. Mostly, people either don't drink it, or they chain-drink it like a crack addict, waking up with their first thought being, "I gotta have me a hit of diet soda." I have ridden my bicycle to the store in my pajamas to get a Diet Coke before I would do anything else. It was ruling my day, every day. And I also know this: I no longer drink diet soda or consume anything with aspartame in it—including chewing gum, candy, or even prescriptions and vaccines—and I don't have migraines anymore. Coincidence? I'm not willing to find out. There's nothing of any value in aspartame that I need. There's no good case for continuing to consume it and a lot of evidence advising against doing so.

I find that getting a monkey off your back is more doable if you can find some replacement. I mean, I wasn't going to go *caffeine*-free on top of ditching the tyrannical NutraSweet. One vice at a time. Unfortunately, some studies suggest that the other artificial sweeteners are probably not much better for you. If you need a sweetener, try honey, molasses, stevia, rice syrup, or sugar (in modest quantities; sugar is better than aspartame but also has its own problems).

If I really feel like partying, I have a regular Coke. But I don't do that too often, because it is made with high-fructose corn syrup, which is genetically modified (and fattening, and of no nutritional value). I may not be Heidi Klum, but I am not ready to have my genes modified—and something tells me consuming genetically modified foods is not going to get me any closer to looking like Heidi.

There are some natural sodas out there, made with juice. And there's seltzer, which is great plain or with a splash of organic juice (read the label, though—some seltzer contains NutraSweet!). I drink a lot of home-brewed green tea with raw honey. Of course, there's always plain water. Remember water? Mankind did pretty well for several eons without sodas to drink.

• • •

Part 3: The Sin of Gluten-y

If I were to take only two steps to improve my autoimmune situation, I would choose these: eliminate excitotoxins (MSG and aspartame) and gluten. What is gluten? It sounds disgusting, so it must be good for you, right? Actually, in this case, no.

Gluten is a hard-to-digest protein found in wheat, rye, spelt, and barley. Gluten intolerance is becoming increasingly common in the United States. More than two hundred symptoms are associated with gluten intolerance, including digestive discomfort, anemia, infertility, osteoporosis, and celiac disease. Food intolerance, as opposed to food allergy, is often overlooked as the possible cause of health problems because the problems caused by food intolerances build up gradually over time. (Food allergies, however, usually make themselves known pretty quickly after eating the offending food.) If it takes weeks or months for the damage to make itself known, how is anyone going to make the connection between the food and the gluten problem?

The simplest way to find out whether a gluten-free diet will benefit you is to try it for two or three weeks and track your symptoms, especially your energy level. There is no risk involved (other than cravings!), and it's something that could possibly make a big difference. Eliminating gluten from my diet has helped me tremendously. Almost every alternative medicine practitioner I have gone to has recommended a gluten-free diet for people with autoimmune diseases.

Unfortunately, gluten seems to be in almost everything: pizza, muffins, bread, cookies, cereal, crackers, soy sauce—even some shampoos! Thankfully, things are much easier now than the first time I went gluten-free. Some restaurants are offering gluten-free menus, and grocery stores offer rice crackers, gluten-free bread, gluten-free cookies, gluten-free pasta, yummy Luna bars, and even rice crust pizza. Of course, the mere fact that something is gluten-free does not mean it is healthy; Tic Tacs are gluten-free, but they're not part of my plan for better health. Eat all processed foods in small quantities.

Here's my secret recipe for homemade gluten-free bread. Start with:

- Bag of Bob's Red Mill Homemade Wonderful GF Bread Mix
- Ingredients listed on back of bag
- One bread machine

Follow the directions on the bag of bread mix. Wait for the bread machine to beep two or three hours later. Hide the bread from everyone else in the house, because it's de-*lish*.

• • •

Part 4: Sodium Nitrate

Sodium nitrate. This chemical is used extensively in meat-packing plants to preserve the meat, so much so that pretty much any meat you buy at your average grocery store or deli is going to have been preserved with sodium nitrate. Is it inflammatory? I'm not sure. Is it toxic? Yes. Large quantities of this chemical have caused cancer in animals.

I sincerely doubt that the average guy behind the deli or meat counter wants to kill you by feeding you something toxic. But did you know that you could kill someone with a large enough dose of sodium nitrate? In fact, a woman who was in love with another woman's husband purposely dosed the wife with sodium nitrate (which she obtained from her job at the meat-packing plant). She gave her enough to make her sick, not kill her. Read about it at www.NaturalNews.com/023873.html.

According to HowStuffWorks.com, stuff like salami, hot dogs, pepperoni, bologna, ham, bacon, and Spam all normally contain sodium nitrate as one of the ingredients. Fresh meats, however, generally do not contain any added chemicals. The chemical is added to inhibit botulism and keep the pink color, so when you open a can of Spam, it's pink instead of gray. (Great—now what am I going to serve on Thanksgiving?)

While it may be unclear whether sodium nitrate is inflammatory, we do know it's toxic. Just ask the wife in the love triangle!

• • •

Part 5: LDL—Luscious Diet of Lard

> *If man made it, don't eat it.*
> **—Jack LaLanne**

LDL (low-density lipoprotein) is the "bad" cholesterol. It increases our body's overall level of inflammation. Inflammation is bad. Thus, LDL is bad. (In contrast, HDL, the "good" cholesterol, seems to be able to remove "bad" cholesterol from the arteries and protect against cardiovascular disease.)

To cut back on LDL, avoid full-fat animal products (fatty meats, cheeses, cream); commercial cakes, cookies, crackers, pies, and breads; refined grains; white bread and potatoes; candy, soda, and sugar, sugar, sugar. Most of us know that we don't need pies and cookies, but you may surprised to learn we also do not need to eat meat or other animal products to be healthy or to get enough protein. On the contrary; according to *Eat to Live*, by Joel Fuhrman, vegetarians live longer and have far less heart disease and cancer. Not only that, pound for pound, broccoli has more protein than steak.

While cutting out all refined sugar won't hurt you, it's not wise to avoid consuming all fat, which would leave you dry-skinned and constipated. (Maybe it is possible to be too thin! Still not sure about the "too rich" thing, though.) It's about eating the right kinds of fat. Good fats actually decrease inflammation.

Where's the good fat? Salmon, nuts, seeds (especially walnuts and flaxseed), fruits, vegetables, and beans (especially soybeans). Yes, fruits and vegetables (and beans) naturally contain fat. Even romaine lettuce has fat in it. Who knew?

The members of the pop band the Archies are probably middle-aged now, and if their eating habits were anything like their number-one hit "Sugar, Sugar," they've probably had to revise their diet, and their lyrics:

> Soybean
> Oh walnut walnut!
> You are my flaxseed girl
> And you got me wanting you

• • •

Part 6: Candida

During my eighteen months on the candida diet, I felt great. This diet involves eating nothing that contains yeast or promotes the growth of *Candida albicans*, a fungus found in the digestive systems of even healthy people. Unfortunately, candida can grow unchecked when your immunity is compromised and thus become a serious health threat. The candida diet is hard: that means virtually no carbohydrates—no wheat, no sugar, no dairy, no chocolate (no reason to live!), not even a piece of fruit. Which is why I nicknamed it the "can't-eat-a" diet, as in "can't eat a dang thing."

Why would I subject myself to this? Because I had thrush (a mushroom farm on my tongue), a not uncommon side effect from taking large doses of prednisone. While I don't think it's a diet I could (or should) ever stick to long-term (our bodies need fruit), the candida diet did rid my system of the yeast overgrowth, and I was at my ideal weight. Best of all, I could go back to sticking my tongue out at the neighbors.

Whether it's on your tongue, in a more embarrassing location, or throughout your system, if you have a yeast overgrowth, this diet, combined with an antifungal medication, will wipe it out. (In addition to embarrassment, candida can also cause inflammation.) You can find out if you have a yeast overgrowth by getting a stool test (and you thought peeing in a jug was gross). Of course, if you have a shiitake crop on your tongue already, you don't need a test to tell you what you already know.

• • •

Part 7: Cut the Cheese

A story I like to refer to as the Case of the Killer Cheese—which I read about in *Food: Your Miracle Medicine*, by Jean Carper— convinced me of just how powerful food really is.

A thirty-eight-year-old British woman had tried everything to deal with her severe rheumatoid arthritis (RA), an autoimmune disease. Finally, some blessed doctor inquired about her cheese cravings, and she admitted to eating as much as a pound of cheese a day. Since she had other allergies in her medical history, they decided to eliminate all dairy products from her diet. Over the next three months, her RA, a disease commonly accepted to be incurable and chronic, completely disappeared.

She accidentally ate some dairy at some point, and her symptoms reappeared. Now the doctors were really curious, so they asked her to try an experiment: she entered the clinic and ate three pounds of cheese, and everyone watched as the RA returned in full force. Twelve days *after stopping* the cheese binge, the symptoms were at their worst.

It takes a while for allergic reactions to food to work their way out of the body, which is why many people never connect the dots between what they eat and the symptoms they experience.

The happy ending is that this woman remains symptom-free as long as she avoids cheese and milk.

There are two kinds of antibodies created by allergic reactions: one causes immediate symptoms, and the other causes delayed onset of symptoms. I already know what gives me hives within a couple of hours of eating it (I'd tell you, but then I'd have to kill you), so when I got a food allergy test, I got the kind where they draw blood and look for delayed reactions. These tests are not always perfect, however. It may be more helpful to go on a "single food rotation diet," as suggested by Steven A. Levine, PhD. On such a diet, no food is eaten more often than once every four days. After four days, the body will either normalize or have such obvious allergic reactions that it will make it hard to deny the problem any longer.

According to Levine in his book *More about Allergy and Addiction*, "Allergy or allergy-like sensitivities nearly always accompany addiction. . . . Allergy may occur without addiction but generally addiction is always accompanied by allergy." In other words, if you are addicted to something—whether it's alcohol, cigarettes, coffee, wheat, sugar, or any other food or substance—you are also allergic to it. Levine says that alcoholics are usually allergic to the grains or yeast used to brew the drink;

coffee addicts are allergic to the coffee bean or the processing chemicals; and habitual smokers are allergic to tobacco and/or the additives.

People with food allergy-addictions, like those addicted to alcohol, coffee, and cigarettes, actually get a little "lift" (or "high") when they consume the food. Then the cravings start as soon as withdrawal symptoms kick in—the kind of cravings that lead you to eat a pound of cheese a day. The problem is that in exchange for that short-term gratification, the body is being forced to deal with an onslaught of offensive substances, and eventually it's going to cause more serious problems than withdrawal, such as our British friend's case of RA.

If it's not clear to you whether you are addicted to something, try giving it up for three weeks. If at first you find yourself tired, achy, crabby, or otherwise uncomfortable, you are addicted. Foods we are allergic/addicted to are usually ones we eat every single day and crave.

Is it worth it to me to avoid a few favorite foods in order to feel better? Well, someone gave up cheese for the rest of her life, and she was British. They have some really nice cheeses in Great Britain!

• • •

Part 8: But I Like Eating Crap!

It can be more work and more expensive to eat well, but according to the Centers for Disease Control, many chronic illnesses are caused by a lousy diet and lack of physical exercise. If you think eating well is expensive and tiresome, and that exercising is inconvenient, try having a chronic illness. The cure for many ills is to simply stop eating and drinking nonfoods.

Yes, some of us have more health problems than we deserve, while others *do* have a lousy diet yet seem never to gain weight or experience other consequences. Most of us know in our hearts, however, that if we want peak performance from our bodies and minds, we should be fueling our bodies with real food, not cartoonish boxes of "fun food."

Will changing my diet increase my odds of living to one hundred? According to *Eat to Live*, by Joel Fuhrman, yes; vegetarians live thirteen years longer than nonvegetarians. (This assumes that these vegetarians are not just replacing animal products with processed carbohydrates, but actually eating fresh vegetables.) We also know that my odds of inflammation are 100 percent if I eat processed foods and lots of animal products, and my odds of heart disease and obesity are quite high. What good is it for modern medicine to keep us alive for one-hundred-plus years if we are riddled with disease?

Forget the hundred-year-old. Eating garbage can even affect those who are young. For example, I know someone who had crazy mood swings when she was a junior in high school. Sometime around her senior year she figured out on her own that sugar and caffeine were causing her mood swings, so she quit drinking caffeine and gave up chocolate. Her grades went up so dramatically that the school invented a Most Improved Student award to recognize the transformation. Was it worth giving up sodas and chocolate bars? You'll have to ask her.

I want to make good choices not because I want to live to be one hundred, because nothing can guarantee that—as the joke goes, "He ate a perfect diet, exercised every day, and got hit by a bus"—but because I want to be healthy, vibrant, and happy for however many years I am on the planet. It's about living well, no matter what age you are.

To prove to myself that I am permanently changing my diet in order to be healthier and not just to be thinner, I stopped weighing myself. If I'm eating a diet of mostly beans and raw, organic fruits and vegetables, my weight will take care of itself. Dieting just to lose weight is about deprivation. Eating to gain health is about getting enough nutrition.

Trust me, I understand that giving up junk food feels like deprivation at first. I'm a reformed crapatarian. But it's like a budget—there are only so many calories you can consume, and

I'd rather "spend" mine on foods that are providing nutrients. Now instead of a diet of mostly inflammatory foods with an occasional salad, I have mostly salad with an occasional (once a week) ounce of cheese or square of chocolate. I love junk food. But I love me more.

• • •

Part 9: Relearning to Eat

The doctor of the future will give no medicine but will interest his patients in the care of the human frame, in diet, and in the cause and prevention of disease.

—Thomas Edison

After we eliminate all that yummy bad stuff, what's left? Lots of things. Most of us eat the same five or ten things over and over, and with the thousands of foods out there, all you have to do is pick another favorite five or ten that are better for you. I discovered the joys of brown rice and beans with green Tabasco sauce, almond butter on rice bread, hummus, avocado with fresh lemon juice, Caesar salad with walnuts, spring mix salad, home-made fruit smoothies, salmon, sweet potatoes, vegetable roll sushi, and Luna bars. Oh, that's eleven—see how easy it is?

To help sort out what foods are "good" and which are "bad," *The Source*, by Woodson Merrell, MD, recommends that you cut back on the "white stuff": salt, sugar, and bleached flour (this means white flour, white rice, white bread, and most pasta). Also, read the labels. If there are more than five ingredients, and you can't pronounce any of them, don't buy that product. Shop around the outside edges of the grocery store. Most of the stuff in the inside aisles is heavily processed food.

When all else fails, use your common sense: "Does this food exist in nature?" If you were stranded in the woods, you would not find Twinkies hanging off bushes or french fries spawning upstream. You'd be eating raw, organic plants, and lots of them. A healthy diet is not just the absence of bad food but the presence of lots of nutritious food.

Want more guidance? Look for one of these diet plans (which are all helpful if you are suffering from a serious illness):

- Gluten free. It's most helpful for those with autoimmune disorders. Read *The G-Free Diet* by Elizabeth Hasselbeck.

- Low-fat vegan. Good for everyone. Vegan means no animal products at all. Need convincing? Don't mind foul language? Read *Skinny Bitch*, by Rory Freedman and Kim Barnouin. Want recipes and testimonials? Read *The Lupus Recovery Diet*, by Jill Harrington.

- Yeast (candida) free. Helpful if you've got an overgrowth of candida. Read *The Candida Diet*, by Helen Gustafson and Maureen O'Shea.

- Whole foods. For a very strict but highly effective diet for everyone, read *Eat to Live*, by Joel Fuhrman. For a book whose author is willing to bargain with you over your favorite vice foods, read the aforementioned *The Source*.

• • •

Chapter 4

Well, Duh! Science Proves Common Sense Right

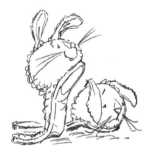

Germs Are Your Friends

"University of Michigan researchers reviewed numerous studies conducted between 1980 and 2006 and concluded that antibacterial soaps that contain triclosan as the main active ingredient are no better than plain soaps," reported *E/The Environmental Magazine*. Not only that, they may pose health risks, such as killing beneficial bacteria and reducing the effectiveness of some antibiotics. (This study was published in the *Journal of Clinical Infectious Diseases*.)

Apparently, triclosan has also been reported to convert into dioxin when exposed to water and UV radiation. Dioxins have been linked to cancer, weakened immunity, decreased fertility, altered sex hormones, and birth defects. In fact, Ukrainian opposition leader Viktor Yushchenko was allegedly poisoned with dioxin and very nearly died. (Do an Internet search for his "before" and "after" pictures. You'll be racing through the house gathering up all the liquid soap to bring to the hazardous-waste dump.) Germs are starting to look less scary all the time, compared to chemicals.

Alcohol-based hand sanitizers are also frowned upon, for stripping the skin of beneficial bacteria and its outer layer of protective oils.

So after all these studies, which probably cost somebody (us?) millions of dollars, what's the best advice?

Washing hands thoroughly for twenty seconds or more with plain soap and warm water is by far the most effective way to reduce harmful bacteria, and as such remains our best defense against getting sick.

—Dairy, Food and Environmental Sanitation, 1998

And the Nobel Prize goes to . . . Captain Obvious!

I have some topics to suggest for their next study: "An apple a day—good or bad?" "Is an ounce of prevention really worth a pound of cure? An updated study using milligrams and kilograms," and "Common sense: a fad?"

Sarcasm aside, it's sad we have to be educated away from all these products that we've been brainwashed into buying. Maybe we really did learn all we needed to know in kindergarten. Okay, that's it. I'm washing my hands of this topic.

• • •

Little Shop of Prayers

Scientists have proven that washing hands with soap kills germs. Shocking, I know. Now they've gone on to prove something else many people already believe: prayer works.

Dr. Franklin Loehr, a Presbyterian minister and scientist, decided to scientifically explore the effectiveness of prayer. In order to avoid the placebo effect (having something work just because the patient believes it is going to work), he used plant seeds. Just to be clear, people prayed for the plant seeds, not the other way around.

This is taking as an assumption that plants do not think. Anyone who has seen *Little Shop of Horrors* might beg to differ, and I, for one, had an African violet that was very fond of Chopin.

But let's play along with Dr. Loehr and say that plants don't think, and therefore they won't know whether or not they're being prayed for.

In one experiment there were three pans of seeds. The first pan received positive prayer, and the second received negative prayer. The third pan, the control pan, was not prayed for at all. The results repeatedly showed that the seeds that were given positive prayer sprouted faster and produced the hardiest plants. The seeds receiving negative prayer did the worst of the three pans. Myself, I've never participated in negative prayer, unless you count that time my mother-in-law put the kibosh on an old boyfriend for me.

After having a stroke, one thing I really appreciated was the huge number of folks all over the country praying for me. I had friends, family, friends of family, family of friends, many of my fans, and several people's entire churches all praying for me. (Thankfully, I hadn't even heard of the concept of "negative prayer" at that point, and I'm pretty sure none of them had either.) Once I found out people were praying for me, it gave me hope. Me, I don't care if the placebo effect wants to try to steal some of the credit. If I know people are praying for me, I feel better already.

Some folks were of different spiritual persuasions and instead offered "positive thoughts" and "healing beams of white light." As long as I was in the first pan of seeds—the ones receiving positive prayer—I was grateful.

Clearly, it worked. You might even say I blossomed.

• • •

Happiness Is Good for You

If a man insisted on being serious and never allowed himself a bit of fun and relaxation, he would go mad or become unstable without knowing it.

—Herodotus

I read a study a while back that said a negative stressor like getting yelled at could negatively affect your immunity for up to twelve hours, whereas a positive experience, such as getting together with friends for fun, can positively affect your immunity for up to three days. It really shouldn't seem like some radical notion that being happy is good for you, but then, people are doing scientific research on the effectiveness of hand washing.

The lesson? It's more important to have fun than it is to avoid stress.

Once I learned about the positive effect of fun on my health, I purposely scheduled regular fun activities to keep myself happy and always have something to look forward to. I set up a reunion with some of my old high school pals, and another with my college pals.

I decided I wanted to join a bicycle club so I could meet folks and have regular social activities (they rode almost every day of the week, and, once I finally joined, I was slower than slow—way behind everybody else in the group—but we all ate at the same table for dinner afterward). I had to work for months just to become strong enough to be the slowest person in the bike club. At the gym, I started on a stationary bike, and I was riding so slowly that the computer cut off; it thought no one was on the bike. So I moved to a bike that had no computer, just a pedal-operated fan. Having the goal of joining the bike club kept me motivated and gave me something to look forward to, and I really enjoyed all the friends I made there.

Some days my fun has to be more low-key than others. When I'm not tracking down old friends from eighth grade or riding a bike at a snail's pace, here are some other things I do for fun:

- Having dinner or a picnic with friends

- Playing games: charades, Farkle, Boggle (the sillier and less competitive, the better)

- Going to the arcade and playing games like Skee-Ball, pinball, and Pac-Man (When I make my millions, I'm putting a Dance Dance Revolution machine in my basement!)

- Shopping at thrift stores

- Swimming

- Watching old sitcoms

- Going to the movies

- Going to weird museums and exhibits (the Beverage Container Museum, the History of Barbed Wire Exhibit)

- Reading comic books

- Writing: journaling, blogging, writing songs, writing parodies

- Turning on some fun music and dancing (goal: look ridiculous)

- Singing

- Making a collage

- Taking a class: tap dancing, stand-up comedy, acting

- Going to camp (There are all kinds of grown-up camps out there now. I've been to songwriting camp and guitar camp. My dad went to a three-day camp and built a canoe, and my mom learned the proverbial—but fun—basket weaving.)

Whatever your favorite flavor of fun is, remember your regular dose of vitamin F!

• • •

Chapter 5

Rubber Chicken Soup: Keeping a Sense of Humor

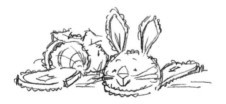

How Can You **Not** Laugh at a Time Like This?

Through humor, you can soften some of the worst blows that life delivers. And once you find laughter, no matter how painful your situation might be, you can survive it.

—Bill Cosby

You can feel so powerless at the doctor's office. You can't get anyone to listen. You can't get them to see you on time. You can't even get them to validate your parking. Illness can steal our energy and our health. Health care can take our time and money. But I'll be darned if they're going to take away my sense of humor.

I was in the hospital at one point and—for some reason—not enjoying myself. Maybe it was the needles. Maybe it was the rubber gloves. Maybe it was the rubber food. All I know is, there's a reason the windows don't open. How else do they keep you from escaping?

About day three of my incarceration, a ray of hope: Saralyn—my bubbliest, silliest friend—called to cheer me up. She jumped from topic to topic, then got to griping about maxipads. I chimed in, complaining about how they stick to everything except what they're supposed to! Next thing you know, I'm writing lyrics about maxipads on a napkin (a dinner napkin, that is). I felt like me again, not just patient 2946065 in bed 31A with diagnosis x, y, and z. I'll always be grateful to Saralyn for that phone call. She not only cheered me up—she brought back my sense of humor.

Spurred on by our marvelous maxipad song creation, I started writing ridiculous songs about everything. The more humiliating, the better. After all, comedy equals pain plus distance, so the more painful it was, the more potentially funny. By falling apart physically, I had haplessly stumbled into a well of comedy gold.

For hours every day, I wrote. I wrote about drug side effects, racing to the bathroom, and even being patient 2946065 in the indigent ward. If it was humiliating or painful, I tried to find the humor in it.

Laughter provides pain relief, lowers blood pressure, boosts the immune system, and even works as exercise—perhaps the only exercise you can get when you're hobbling around with a cane. Just as importantly, it gave me my power back. If you've ever been to a comedy club, you know the funny person in the room is the one with all the power. She can speak the truth, and she can make people listen to her. It also changed the way I looked at and felt about what was happening to me. I started seeing the world through laugh-colored lenses. Once I stepped back and saw the absurdity of my situation, I really had to say, "How can you *not* laugh at a time like this?"

"The Maxipad Song"
(Sing to the tune of "My Favorite Things")

I'm cranky and crampy, my jeans are too tight

I'm looking for comfort, not for a flight

I just want the confidence maxis will bring

The kind that do not have those stupid old wings

When the curse strikes

When the flow comes

When I'm feeling bad

I don't want those wings sticking to everything

I just want a plain old pad

• • •

Funny or Not

Let's face it, most folks are uncomfortable around sick people. They don't know what to say, and they're scared. We sure could use a laugh right about then, but no one, including the patient, knows what to say or do. How do we know what's funny and what's not in this situation? It's kinda like this:

- Getting a painful bone marrow test? Not funny. Wearing SpongeBob SquarePants underwear to the appointment? Funny.

- Lying in the hospital bed while a bunch of doctors talk about you as if you're not there? Not funny. Setting up a fart machine at the foot of your bed? Funny.

- You making jokes about my illness? Not funny. Me making jokes about my illness? Funny.

- You making jokes about my illness while wearing a funny nose and glasses? Still not funny! You telling me you fell down a manhole on the way to come visit me? Funny.

Remember, comedy is pain plus distance. So if it's happening to me right now, and it's painful, I may not be ready to laugh about it. I probably really *need* to laugh about *something*, but to be safe, let's choose a topic other than my health problems (like, for instance, your problems, how bad the art on the hospital wall is, or which celebrity just got their worst mugshot ever).

Comedy involves pain, and that pain needs a target, so let's aim it at someone other than the person already in pain. Even if I make a little joke about my own situation, that is not an invitation for everyone else to pile on and start making jokes about it, anymore than it would be okay for people who are not Hispanic to make fun of Hispanic people or who are not Jewish to make fun of Jews. You have permission to mock your own situation, but mocking others' situation is insensitive. And even worse: not funny.

• • •

Take Two Movies and Call Me in the Morning

A merry heart doeth good like a medicine but bitterness rots the bones.

—Proverbs 15:13

Humor has been getting a lot of serious attention among researchers in the last decade, due in part to Norman Cousins's book *Anatomy of an Illness*, as well as the efforts of Dr. Patch Adams and organizations like the Association for Applied and Therapeutic Humor. The research is proving what we've known all along: laughter is good for your health, stress is tough on your system, your outlook on life affects your physical well-being, and having a sense of humor makes you more resilient.

When Norman Cousins was given little chance of surviving his illness (Marie-Strumpell disease) and no drug was able to relieve him of his pain, he discovered that ten minutes of genuine belly laughter provided him two hours of pain-free sleep. Three Stooges movies relieved him of the pain that no narcotic could ease. Once the effect of the laughter wore off, he'd turn on the movie again.

In 2005 researchers at the University of Maryland published a humor study titled *The Impact of Cinematic Viewing on Endothelial Function*. That's fancy talk for "a bunch of heart patients got to watch movies as part of their treatment." I think I can safely say they were out to scientifically prove what Norman Cousins had discovered: laughter is the best medicine, and movies are a great delivery system for laughs.

The findings? Viewing a comedy movie led to a 22 percent increase in blood flow, while viewing a stressful film led to a 35 percent decrease. The effects lasted thirty to forty minutes. The people in the comedy video group had fewer recurrent heart attacks and lower blood pressure.

All this expensive research and fancy vocabulary just goes to show what we knew all long: a merry heart really *does* doeth good like a medicine.

There is one hitch, however: subsequent attempts to replicate the trial results were inconsistent because they did not differentiate between positive and negative humor. Just as a well-honed positive sense of humor doeth good like a medicine, a well-honed negative sense of humor doeth bad like a poison.

If you are ready to do your heart good like a medicine, or, if you prefer, "enjoy the improved endothelial function derived from cinematic viewing," rent yourself some funny movies or read the funnies. Or tune into some old sitcoms on Nick at Nite instead of watching people getting attacked and killed on *Law and Order*. If you're trying to figure out the difference between positive and negative humor, go for goofy, light, silly, and fun (think vaudeville, slapstick, Disney, Jim Carrey, *I Love Lucy*, *SpongeBob SquarePants*). Avoid sarcastic and mean (racist or sexist humor, or anything that tears other people down or focuses on complaining).

Patch Adams recommends the following in his book *Gesundheit!*: Charlie Chaplin, Buster Keaton, W. C. Fields, the Marx Brothers, the Three Stooges, Laurel and Hardy, Abbott and Costello, Lucille Ball, Red Skelton, Jonathan Winters, Sid Caesar, Carol Burnett, Ernie Kovacs, Jerry Lewis, Woody Allen, Lily Tomlin, Monty Python, PeeWee Herman, and *Saturday Night Live*.

Here are ten of my favorite funny movies: *Honey I Shrunk the Kids, Aladdin, The Incredibles, Toy Story, Monsters, Inc., Shrek, Mrs. Doubtfire, Dirty Rotten Scoundrels, Some Like It Hot, Ruthless People*.

If you're looking for funny movies, the American Film Institute and Bravo have both compiled lists of the top one hundred funny movies of all time. Some of the movies on those lists are not really laugh-out-loud funny (such as *The Graduate* or most Woody Allen movies), but they are a good place to start. Netflix and Blockbuster have comedy categories you can browse through, as does any video store. Some local libraries even have

movies you can check out for free. Having trouble picking something out? I really like www.theseriouscomedysite.com, as it
gives lots of details on and reviews of funny movies, CDs,
books, and comedians. Take two movies and reel in the laughs.

• • •

Give a Man a Rubber Chicken, and He'll Laugh for a Day

Give a man a fish, and you feed him for a day. Teach a man to fish, and you feed him for a lifetime.

—Chinese proverb

I love this quote because it's a life lesson in only two sentences, and I love the lesson: teaching someone to be independent, helping them to help themselves, is in the end a much greater gift than simply giving them handouts.

I try to do this as a guitar teacher. I could just teach my students a bunch of songs, but if they didn't understand what they were doing, they'd be helpless without someone there to keep spoon-feeding them songs. So I teach them a little theory, how to read notation, and how things move around on the guitar. My ultimate success as a teacher is when they come to the point where they can figure things out for themselves and no longer need me. Give a guitar student a song, and he'll play for three minutes. Teach him to play guitar, and he'll entertain himself for hours on end. And spend all his disposable income on musical instruments. But I digress.

After hearing about all the health benefits of laughter, and all the detrimental effects of stress and negative outlook, I got to thinking. Tell a man a joke, and he'll laugh for a minute. Teach him how to laugh, and he'll be amused for a lifetime.

I wondered: But what if you just can't tickle the guy's funny bone? What if you can't figure out what makes him laugh? How can we help someone who just isn't easily amused?

Then I learned about the World Laughter Club. Through a series of exercises, they teach people how to laugh on cue, and they organize events where people gather and laugh together. Even if they are just going through the motions and not laughing at anything in particular, they are still getting all the physical benefits of laughter, including relaxation, reduction of stress chemicals (corticoids and epinephrine), and an overall improved sense of well-being. Once you get past the initial "I feel like an idiot," you've got a great tool at your disposal.

Even the most humor-impaired person can still learn to laugh every single day if she so chooses—even the guy who sits in the audience at a comedy club and yells, "You suck!" at the performer. (And while the heckler may be right—maybe the comedian really *does* suck—would you rather be right or would you rather be laughing?)

• • •

Chapter 6

Take a Mind off Your Load: Expressing Yourself and Keeping It Positive

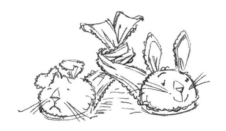

The Three Faces of Me

Some folks say autoimmune disease has a thousand faces. What they mean is that it resembles so many other medical problems that it can be hard to diagnose. Once you've got a chronic illness, you feel like you yourself have a thousand faces, or at least three: one for the public (I'm fine), one for the doctor (I'm sick), and one for home (I'm me). It's a lot to keep up with! These are my three faces:

The Public Face

In public I just want to be treated like a normal person. I don't want everyone staring at me, whispering about me, treating me like I'm made of glass. Basically, I'd like to not be reminded of my problems at every turn. When I go out with friends, I want to talk about something else, anything else.

The Patient's Face

Then I go to the doctor, and if I don't look sick, he doesn't take me seriously. I don't wear makeup to the doctor or spend a lot of time on my hair that day. (Not that I spend much time on it anyway, unless it's a big occasion.) I definitely don't dress *up* for the doctor, no matter how hot he is. He needs to see my complexion as it is naturally, because my illness causes redness, acne, rashes, and lesions, and anemia causes paleness. This, of course, is the stuff I hide for face number 1.

While I work hard not to focus on my problems and try not to keep in the forefront of my mind a list of my aches and pains and diagnoses, I can't show up to the doctor and say, "Oh, I'm fine" (unless I am!). You only get five minutes with the guy, so you have to write down your problems somewhere, then be able to rattle them off when you see him so he can have some record of symptoms, in case there's a pattern. If you don't list your problems, he can't treat them. If you don't ask for help and mention your pain, you can't be surprised when your pain isn't properly managed. But, again, I don't want to think about it more than I have to.

After the doctor visit, I try to wipe off that disease-centered mind-set once I get in the car. Then I put on face number 1 (public face) until I get home and can put on face number 3.

My Real Face

Sometimes faces 1 and 2 can leave me confused about what my real face is. Who am I? A person with autoimmune disease who is hiding it, or just trying to live with it? A person who is minimizing, exaggerating, ignoring, or complaining about it? Maybe I'm an otherwise interesting person who just happens to have this health thing going on. Maybe I'm just a person with a problem.

I try to remember who I am/was before the diagnosis. I find "me" when I'm able to lose myself doing things I love, such as creating music, writing songs, writing blogs, joking around with friends, laughing myself silly, playing with the dog, or creating anything.

I believe if we're made in the image of the Creator, then we must be made to create. When we create things or are creative, we are being the most like God. For some folks, that's visual arts and crafts, or cooking, or improvisation. For me, it's composing music or writing. Whether you feel that way or not, I do find that doing anything I love—even if I'm just laughing my head off—makes me feel like "me."

That's my third face, the childlike, honest face, what some would call my essence: the face that isn't thinking at all about what it looks like to other people, and is just being.

What are your faces?

• • •

Designer Labels

How do you refer to yourself when you have a serious chronic illness? Say, for example, I had the plague. What would I call myself? Plague patient? Depersonalizing. Plague victim? Definitely not. Plaguey? Um, no. Person with the plague? Sounds like a police suspect. Plague survivor? Sounds like I'm over it. (Not yet.) Plague warrior? A little too dramatic.

After I recovered from my first bout with chronic illness, I would say, "I had an autoimmune disease, but I don't anymore." Subsequent experiences have certainly humbled me enough to not want to use that verbiage again. Words matter, and they matter a lot. Since I hold my own opinion in higher esteem than just about anyone else's, when I say something, and hear myself say it, I take it to heart. So now I want to carefully choose how I describe my situation. Sometimes I say, "I've been diagnosed with autoimmune disease." It's a little clunky, but it's closer to how I feel.

Even more than a decade after being diagnosed, I just can't stomach saying out loud, "I have a chronic disease." That has a real finality to it and sounds to me like I've accepted that it will always be there, all day, every day for the rest of my life. I don't want disease to be a headline in my life. I can just hear the eulogy: "Disease disease disease. And then she died. Of disease." If illness has to be mentioned, I want it to receive only a footnote in my life story. I need a phrase that gives more power to me and less to the illness.

I'm taking a cue from Jenny McCarthy, who wrote a book about her remarkable and inspiring experience as the mother of a child with autism. While she hesitates to say that her son is healed, because she feels that his autism could be retriggered by environmental and dietary toxins, she does say he is recovered. I think maybe that's a label I could live with: recovering. Like a recovering alcoholic: "I'm recovering from autoimmune disease." Then I'm acknowledging the problem (and the need to be vigilant) without surrendering to it and letting it become my identity, or my destiny.

Yeah, I'm recovering from several autoimmune diseases. And I'm also a guitar player, a songwriter, a teacher, an aunt, a wife, a daughter, a dog owner, a friend, a marching band geek, a gardener, a lover of words, smart, a little zany, and kinda cute.

• • •

Can You Hear Me Now?

I was at a songwriters' retreat some years ago, and I was wondering: why have so many people become songwriters? It seems like everybody has a CD or a band, or writes songs. Is it a movement? A seeking of truth? The second coming of the "great folk scare" of the sixties that would rise up and change the world with its protest songs?

I asked this very question of another songwriter, a deep thinker and great songwriter whom I respect a lot and who had attained a somewhat notable level of success. I braced myself for some of his profound, meaningful, spiritual wisdom, and he said, "It's because it's so cheap to make CDs now."

I climbed to the top of the mountain to see the guru, and this is what I got? Well, I guess even the guru has an off day. So after a decade of mulling this over myself, I think I now know why so many people are writing songs and making CDs: the only way people can express themselves and get other people to listen is by turning it into art.

People no longer have any chance to tell their story. There is no oral tradition, no passing on of the old stories while sitting on the porch or around the fire. I once started to tell a six-year-old a story about when I was a kid, and she screamed, *"I don't want to listen!"* Wow. Well, the TV *was* on. (Then again, the TV is always on, everywhere you go.)

All most of us want is to be seen, heard, and loved for who we are, but no one seems to want to listen.

I, for one, became a songwriter because I was incapable of directly telling people how I really feel. If I had something I needed to discuss with a boyfriend, he'd have to hear me singing it through the wall of the music practice room. I'm much better at communicating with my husband, which is part of the reason I married him, but I still struggle to communicate with the rest of the world. I write songs because I have something I need to say, and that seems to be the only way I can say it. It's the same reason people paint, sculpt, write books, and dance. It's also the reason some hospitals offer art therapy, music therapy, and even creative writing therapy—people need to express themselves.

That, in my opinion, is why there are so many songwriters out there. Sure, it's cheap and easy to make a CD, but it's also cheap and easy to go jump off a bridge. Writing songs and making art in general is an act of hope, of finding ourselves and reaching out to others to connect, to try one more time to find someone who will hear us.

• • •

Obecalp: The Miracle Drug!

The best and most efficient pharmacy is within your own system.

—Robert C. Peale, MD

Obecalp is the gold standard against which all other drugs are measured. If a drug cannot outperform Obecalp in a trial, it will not be approved for use. It's consistently effective in 33 percent of patients for all kinds of ailments, and it's incredibly cheap.

Strangely, Obecalp only has whatever side effects the patient expects it to have, and it is only as effective as the patient believes it is. It is a pill that allows us to harness the power of the mind to heal our bodies. Doctors order Obecalp from the pharmacy when they have no other available treatment for the ailment. What the heck is Obecalp? It's *placebo* spelled backward. It's a sugar pill. A placebo is a pill that has no actual drug in it, but is presented to the patient as if it were a therapeutic drug. The patient thinks it is a drug, and for that reason alone, it has a therapeutic effect on 33 percent of patients.

The one thing that renders Obecalp completely ineffective is telling the patient that it's a placebo. Too bad, because I'd much rather take a harmless sugar pill than pretty much any of the drugs I've been prescribed. Wouldn't it be great if I could ask for the placebo, then somehow not know it was a placebo? I need a doctor who can do Jedi mind tricks. Of course, I'd have to trust such a powerful doctor, and that's another topic entirely. So since I can't ask for a placebo and have it work, and I don't know any doctors who are also trustworthy Jedi knights (they can always go to the dark side), this leaves me on the hunt for some other way to harness the power of my own mind to heal my body. This is why I find it cruel to tell patients that something that is working for *them*—prayer, acupuncture, herbs, homeopathy—is "only" psychosomatic, all in their head. That is stealing not only their hope, but their actual healing.

During my second bout with autoimmune diseases, I had a pair of small strokes (TIAs) and I couldn't use my left hand or get up and down even one stair. I had an acupuncturist who was treating me almost every day. She told me that all day, every day, our minds send "live" and "die" messages to the rest of our being. I needed to be more cognizant of what kind of messages I was sending myself, or all the effort she was putting into treating me was just going to evaporate.

I was later told something similar by another acupuncturist, who was treating me for an extremely negative emotional reaction to Novocain. I would always feel better after the treatment, but within a matter of hours I would be moody and depressed again. She finally said, "You have to hang on to your treatment." I didn't like disappointing her, so I was determined not to show up at her office having had her treatment evaporate again. When I started to feel the bad moods trying to take me over again, I would tell them, "No. I am not going there." I realized I was able to choose which thoughts I paid attention to.

I can't break down for you exactly how this works, but it does. The body-mind connection is well documented. Don't believe me? Here's a simple example. Think about a lemon, and saliva develops in your mouth at just the memory of the lemon's tart taste.

We make little "life" and "death" decisions all day, every day, not just in what we eat and how much rest we get, but in which thoughts we choose to focus on and which feelings we allow to dominate us. I don't have to be tricked into feeling better with sugar pills and Jedi mind tricks; I can consciously choose life.

Note: To find more information on the body-mind connection, look for books under the fancy scientific names "biopsychosocial" and "psychoneuroimmunology."

• • •

What I Learned by Being a Lousy Athlete

Although the world is full of suffering, it is also full of the overcoming of it.

—Helen Keller

I've always been a below-average athlete. I was often picked last at recess and generally had to work really hard to be even average in any sport. The great thing about doing things that you're not very good at is that it offers a great opportunity to learn—about self-mastery, humility, persistence, and other life lessons.

The first and only time I went mountain biking, the trail was muddy and very narrow, with a steep drop-off on one side. After falling off the bike once, all I could think about was falling off the bike again. There were many obstacles in the path, such as tree roots and rocks. I'd see them coming and stare at them, terrified of falling off the bike, and sure enough, that's exactly what happened. About twelve times. Finally, I got off the bike and walked the rest of the trail.

Later that year, I ended up going on a ski trip with some friends. (Maybe I thought winter would be less hazardous than summer, or maybe I just forgot how uncoordinated I can be.) Whenever I started moving too fast, my strategy was to purposely fall over so I could stop. That was working fine until I saw the snow machine (which was cranking out tons of icy stuff), and I thought, "Oh, let me land anywhere except there." So, of course, staring at the snow machine, I was drawn to it like a moth to a flame, like a deer in the headlights, like flies to. . . . Well anyway, I fell right in front of it and got plastered in snow and ice.

What I learned from all this was the importance of focusing on where you *want* to go, rather than where you're afraid you might end up. If I were to look for openings instead of obstacles, I would have biked and skied through the open spaces instead of ramming right into the obstacles. Fear is just faith in reverse— strong belief in a bad outcome rather than a good one.

After my strokes, I got an opportunity to put this belief into action. I had lost the ability to play the guitar, but I refused to accept that I might never play again. Instead of even allowing that thought to take hold, I focused instead on where I wanted to go: I wanted to be able to play guitar as well as I ever did. Once in a while the thought "What if I never play again?" would enter my head, and I would reject it. I refused to even entertain that "what if," because that was my snow machine at the bottom of the hill: exactly where I did not want to end up. So every time such a thought would enter my head, I'd say, "I am going to play as well as I ever did, maybe even better," and I would picture it.

Meanwhile, the process of getting where I wanted to be was slow, but if it were easy, I wouldn't need to have faith. Attempting to play the guitar was extremely painful—because of the neuropathy (nerve pain), just touching the strings felt like needles were being stuck into my fingertips. I tried gluing corn pads on my fingertips and using those rubber tips that cashiers put on their fingers. It sort of worked, but because of the stroke, my left hand was too weak to apply enough pressure to get the notes to sound good. So I looked for an opening.

I've taught little kids with no hand strength to play guitar—you just have to get a friendly enough instrument. So I went on eBay and bought myself a ukulele for eight bucks. The uke has finger-friendly nylon strings, and they require a lot less left-hand strength to get good notes. It worked! I was making music again!

I later graduated to a larger ukulele and eventually regained my guitar playing entirely, just as I had pictured. Now to conquer that ski slope . . .

• • •

Survivor: Kidney Island

If you watch the "reality" show *Survivor*, you'll walk away thinking that in order to survive, you need to lie, scheme, manipulate, and backstab. This approach is of no help at all, however, when you're trying to survive an illness. It might make for good TV, but it makes for horrible life lessons.

When I was uninsured and forced to go to an indigent kidney clinic, I was living my own survivor series. In one particularly riveting episode, one of the doctors (whom I saw once) told me that I'd need a kidney transplant and/or dialysis within five years. Then he swiftly got up and left the room while I tried to process this prognosis.

I've known several people who have received dialysis. It's life-saving, but it's a big commitment. Once you start treatment, you're usually on it for life or until you get a kidney transplant. And I was only in my thirties. You can't lie or backstab your way out of a situation like that, and there is no "immunity idol" to spare you. You have to actually stand up and fight. I cried for about an hour. Then I said, "This is unacceptable. I will not accept this." And I started to fight.

I knew from my previous ten years of living with this illness that doctors don't know everything, and that we can beat the odds if we have the tools. I also knew that if I accepted his prognosis, I would resign myself to the situation and not try to improve it. It would become a self-fulfilling prophecy.

From everything I had read about the body-mind connection, I believed that I had a choice in the outcome. I've always been fascinated by stories of people who survived things like plane crashes and weeks in lifeboats while everyone else around them perished. How did they do it? In many cases, they made a conscious decision at a crucial moment to survive. I knew if I made the choice to survive, I could beat his prognosis. Why did I believe I could be one of the "lucky" ones?

Among other things, it was something I read in Bernie Siegel's book *Love, Medicine and Miracles*. Even though he is an oncologist, the principles he shares about healing apply to anyone with any illness. One paragraph that made me jump out of my chair was the one that describes what makes an exceptional patient—one who beats the odds. According to Bernie, a survivor:

- Is good at what she does for a living and enjoys it

- Is sometimes hostile

- Has a strong ego

- Retains control of his life

- Is receptive and intelligent

- Has a strong sense of reality

- Is self-reliant

- Is nonconformist

- Seeks solutions and doesn't see problems as failures

- Makes use of her time in the waiting room rather than staring into space

Luckily for me, the self-reliance, intelligence, and nonconformity came naturally. (As did the occasional hostility.) I had to work at some of the others, especially not seeing the illness as a personal failure.

Speaker/author/patient C. W. Metcalf boiled down the traits of survivors to five: humor, altruism, community, imagination, and divinity.

The great news is, even if you don't have any of these attributes, you can develop them. You can *become* a survivor. It's one of the greatest lessons an illness can teach you.

As for me? So far, so good. It's been more than five years since that prognosis, and I have full kidney function—and both of my own original kidneys. I also gained an immunity idol— knowing the traits of a survivor—that I can use over and over for the rest of my life.

• • •

Platitude of Gratitude

Everything can be taken from a man but one thing: the last of the human freedoms—to choose one's attitude in any given set of circumstances, to choose one's own way.
—Viktor E. Frankl, *Man's Search for Meaning*

"Attitude of gratitude." I've always hated that phrase. Someone said that to me a long, long time ago when I was feeling particularly sorry for myself for some reason. At the time I felt that my self-pity was entirely justified and that, indeed, my life was worse than anyone else's on the planet.

In such a moment, the last thing you want to hear is, "You need to get an attitude of gratitude." If you're me, your immediate reaction is, "Attitude of gratitude? Cram it with your stupid platitude! How can you be thankful when everything stinks?"

When I developed autoimmune disease several years later, I learned the true meaning of "everything stinks." I could not work, eat, or even care for myself, and I had a fever that spiked to 104°F every afternoon.

Someone from the church said to me, "You need to rejoice in the Lord." I wanted to kick his ass! Of course, I couldn't even get off the couch on my own, so he was safe. But, really, I mean, what did he know about my pain? Nothing! My life was a mess, and his was fine.

Rejoice in the Lord? Are you kidding me? What was I supposed to do? Jump up and down? Dance? Sing? I wasn't physically capable at that time of doing any of those things—I had even lost most of my voice.

I was right—my life was crap at that point. But *he* was also right—there were still things to be grateful for, and choosing gratitude would have at least lifted the burden off my soul, if not my body. I just couldn't bridge that chasm between despair and joy. I didn't know how.

Yet, somewhere along the way I learned how to cultivate an attitude of gratitude, for which, yes, I am thankful. You can learn to be thankful, even if it's not in your nature, and you can change your attitude, even if you don't think of yourself as a sunny person. One very simple tool can help you do this: make a gratitude list.

Now, even something as simple as making a daily list of five things you're thankful for seems preposterous when you are in constant pain, your hair is falling out, your bank account is being drained by medical expenses, you've lost your job because of your illness, and you've been robbed of your youth and independence at age twenty-five. But it all comes down to this: would you rather be right or be happy? Yes, you have a right to be sad. Yes, you could wallow in self-pity. But at some point, after we've had a moment to feel our feelings, we have to dust ourselves off, be thankful anyway, and say, "There are good things in my life. I want to put my focus on those good things instead of the bad."

Choosing to give thanks is something that will help *you*. Your nurse, your friends, your spouse, your mom, and certainly your higher power or God are going to get along okay whether or not you say thank-you. They are happy to hear it and probably deserve to hear it, but the focus at this moment is you.

Having a grateful heart turns you from a downward spiral of pain and self-pity into an upward spiral of gratitude and possibility. It's a slow, gradual process, not instant gratification, but it's worth it. Becoming grateful as a habit yields long, deep results. When you look for what's good, you start noticing more good things, and that gradually changes the habit of complaining to one of celebrating.

Now, I'm not going to tell you what to be grateful for, because that's annoying and presumptuous. I still fall into occasional pits of self-pity, and I usually remember at some point that I need to start making a daily gratitude list. The first list is always the hardest to compile, because I've gotten back into the habit of looking at everything that's wrong. So I start as small as I have to. Like: I'm thankful my house has heat. I'm thankful I have hair. I'm thankful for my dog. I'm thankful I have a car that works. I'm thankful I have a TV to watch when I can't sleep. I'm thankful for good music. I'm thankful for heating pads. I'm thankful for Icy Hot (which you should never use in combination with heating pads). I'm thankful I have pain medication. I'm thankful for my friends. I'm thankful for the Internet, where I can type to someone when all my friends are asleep.

The next thing you know, I've written three pages of things in my life that I'm grateful for. I'm thankful ballpoint pens are so cheap.

• • •

Wax On, Wax Off, Wax Philosophical

The life unexamined is not worth living.

—Plato

I never thought I'd say this, but I really like kung fu movies. Add this to my love of the Rocky movies (minus *Rocky IV*) and my ability to burp on command, and, well, you'd never believe my name translates as "feminine."

My husband has studied martial arts for more than a decade, and long ago, pre–chronic illness, I did about six months' training in American karate. I never got very good at fighting since we never practiced sparring. I did take second place in a sparring tournament—out of two people. I got creamed. ("Point! Point! Point!" "What happened?") Ah well, I'm pretty much a pacifist anyway, I told myself.

Okay, so I like Jackie Chan. Who doesn't? That's like saying, "I like pizza." After my husband made me watch *The Last Dragon* (no words to describe how awful), that was it: no more kung fu movies for me! Then I saw a copy of *Kung Fu Hustle* in the thrift shop and bought it as a joke for my hubby. I figured if he liked *The Last Dragon*, he'd love this. It sounded horrible—right up his alley!

To my shock and amazement, it was fabulous! We then watched all four *Karate Kid* movies, Jet Li's *Fearless, Shaolin Soccer*, and *Forbidden Kingdom*, all of them wonderful. The good kung fu movies all seem to not only have incredible feats of athleticism, but people who have a depth of honor, character, and self-possession that can come only from years of study and self-discipline.

Aside from stumbling upon Stephen Chow, what changed my mind entirely about kung fu is learning from my husband that *kung fu* means "time and effort." You discover yourself and master yourself (and therefore, your world) through the deep study of . . . almost anything.

I realized that writing is my kung fu. I learn about myself through songwriting, blogging, journaling, and even composing letters to friends. I pour myself into my writing, and it reflects to me what I need to know. Through writing I've learned to look for the deeper meaning in everything, to read between the lines, and to look for the divine or the spiritual in everything. Your kung fu holds the key to life's lessons for you.

My husband's martial arts teacher says, "What you struggle with in kung fu, you struggle with in life." If you struggle with balance, flexibility, or allowing yourself to be ruled by fear when you are sparring, you are probably struggling with these things in the rest of your life, too.

Recovering from a serious illness is going to require much time and much effort, and for this reason, it can become your teacher (your kung fu) while it is in your life. What may have seemed to be a horrible curse at first may turn out to be an opportunity to learn more about yourself, what you value, and your relationship to the world.

• • •

What's Free?

Here's a lesson from martial arts that translates well to dealing with illness: what's free? No, I don't mean who's giving away free drug samples. I mean, when it seems like you're pinned down by your opponent, *what's free* to fight back with?

Now granted, I don't have a lot of martial-arts experience, but it seems to me if someone's got you in a headlock, with the "what's free?" mind-set, you think, "Hey, his arms are busy holding my head—but mine are free! I could punch him in the kidney, pull his leg hair, give him a wedgie, or grab his testicles." He'd let go of your head at some point.

I love this lesson because it helps refocus from your seeming limitations to whatever possibilities might still be open. You start to brainstorm and get really creative. It's a great kick-start to getting into a solution-oriented frame of mind. It's easy to say, "Be solution oriented!" But how do you start doing that? By asking, "What's free?"

Several years back I was watching an infomercial for Richard Simmons, whom I love. (Suddenly I have no room to pick on my husband's taste in movies.) Richard's message is simple: get moving!

The infomercial was filled with testimonials of folks who had lost weight, some of them a hundred pounds or more. But what really grabbed me was the girl in the wheelchair. I don't remember why she was in a wheelchair, but I do remember that she had been there for years, and she was probably always going to be in a wheelchair. And she got Richard Simmons's exercise videos and exercised in her wheelchair.

She didn't wait for Richard to make a video especially for someone in a wheelchair, nor did she say, "Everyone in the video is walking and kicking, and I can't do that." Instead she said, "What's free?" and she moved her upper body, and she sweated, got stronger, and lost weight.

When my legs were too weak to walk after I had a stroke, what was free? My arms were getting pretty strong from dragging the rest of me around with no help from my legs. I could swim like a fish with those strong arms! And eventually, I got the strength back in my legs.

I had also lost the strength in my left hand, but I'm right-handed, so I could still write. I also still had a sense of humor, so I wrote parodies—I took existing songs and wrote new lyrics to them. All the songs were humorous and about irritating medical stuff I was dealing with: "Prednisone," "Sittin' in the Waiting Room," "On the Commode Again," and "What If Your Butt Was Gone." I ended up with an entire CD of humorous medical songs. I called it "Sick Humor."

It was cathartic—anytime a doctor made me mad, I'd write a song. Instead of staying trapped by my limitations, I kept saying, "What's free?"

• • •

The T-shirt I'm Not Going to Buy

We have been taught to believe that negative equals realistic and positive equals unrealistic.

—Susan Jeffers

I get really tired of explaining myself to those people who view me as just lazy rather than as someone with a chronic illness. However, I refuse to buy a T-shirt that says, I HAVE LUPUS. WHAT'S YOUR EXCUSE?

I understand firsthand how frustrating it is to be exhausted and in constant pain and to have people telling you your problems aren't real. However, the day I start wearing that kind of T-shirt, I know I've given in and gone to the dark side, where I define myself by my illness and become a perpetual victim. Where I talk about my illness to anyone who will listen, and many who won't, and spend more energy defending my right to be sick and getting other people to feel sorry for me than I do living my life to its full potential. Word to the wise: usually you're not very interesting or fun to be around when your whole world is your illness.

Once when I was in the hospital, I ran into the chaplain, whom I had met the day before, and she said, "Oh, I remember you. You're lupus." I was too offended to speak. I am *not* a disease! I am a person! She may as well have called me Satan.

Another time I was at a friend's house in South Carolina. This friend also had a serious illness. Her son was making us dinner. I was coming along well in my recovery, and I even had a little energy. In my usual spirit of doing as much as I was able to for myself, I started toward the kitchen and offered to help out. My friend whispered to me, "Stop! You're ruining it!" I was shocked. She had plenty of valid excuses to do absolutely nothing, but it felt like she was using her illness to make her son do all the housework. She was choosing helplessness, at least to some degree. Anyone with a diagnosis of a serious or chronic illness has a great excuse to just rest. But I don't want an excuse—I want a life.

I don't identify myself by my illness, and I certainly am not going to invite others to do so by wearing my diagnosis on my chest like either a scarlet letter or a badge of honor. So instead of a T-shirt saying, I HAVE LUPUS. WHAT'S YOUR EXCUSE? I ordered one that says, I ♥ CARLA.

• • •

Get Busy Living or Get Busy Dying

Every time you don't follow your inner guidance, you feel a loss of energy, loss of power, a sense of spiritual deadness.

—Shakti Gawain

In Bernie Siegel's book *Love, Medicine and Miracles*, he asks his patients what their lives were like for the year before they got sick. In my case, I had squashed myself down into a life that wasn't making me happy—getting up early six days a week and putting on a suit, panty hose, and heels to go to a minimum-wage job I hated. I spent the seventh day (again in suit, hose, and heels) attending a church where I didn't fit in. I was living in a town I didn't like, in a house that should have been condemned. Once the landlord got rid of the roaches, we got ants, then slugs, then camel crickets.

Let me take a moment to explain how disgusting camel crickets are. They look like a mix between a grasshopper and a daddy longlegs, they can hop across a room, and they bite. They like to hang out in the shower, and when you kill them, they leave bloodstains. Every morning I took a flip-flop into the bathroom and killed about eight camel crickets before I could get in the shower. Excuse me for a sec; I think I have a plot idea for a sequel to *Psycho*.

My diet wasn't anything to brag about, either. I drank a liter of diet soda a day, and since I worked for minimum wage, I ate as cheaply as possible, often having a 50-cent candy bar for breakfast and something from the Taco Bell (aka "Toxic Smell") 69-cent menu for lunch. Is this a recipe for health?

When I got too sick to care for myself, I lost my job and spent my savings. I had to start all over. Once I got back on my feet (literally), I fashioned myself a life that was worth living. If you don't learn anything else from surviving a near-death experience such as stroke or kidney failure, hopefully you learn that you only live once. And if you hate everything in your life, you realize you've got a second chance to rebuild your life from scratch, only this time on purpose.

As the Tim Robbins character said in *The Shawshank Redemption*, "Get busy living or get busy dying."

I decided to do what I was good at and what I loved doing: teaching guitar in my own studio and writing songs. Now I was self-employed doing meaningful work with plenty of time to be creative. I gave myself Saturdays off. My new boss (me) paid me more than minimum wage. And I never wore panty hose again.

In some respects, the dream of having a teaching studio was a modest one—it wasn't like sending a man to the moon or building a real estate empire. But in another respect it was as big and courageous a dream as any person can have: the dream of being true to myself and using my gifts—the only kind of dream that ever really makes anyone happy.

Will following my heart save me from ever getting sick again? Who knows, it might. Some folks with a terminal diagnosis decide to go out and start making the most of their last days, then end up fully recovering. More likely, it is just one piece of the puzzle in what it takes to get and stay well.

Either way, I win. If I get sick again, I have a life worth fighting for. If I stay well, I have a life worth living.

Things to Do Before I Die— Why Wait?

Part of creating a life worth living is having dreams (aka a "bucket list," or a list of things to do before you die), and then fulfilling those dreams. My list of things to do before I die just got shorter by one huge event. I finally got to see Van Halen, the original Van Halen (with David Lee Roth, their original singer). I understand that not everyone thinks of a loud, raucous rock concert of screaming guitar and a glib, vulgar, egomaniacal front man as utopia, but I do.

If you're not a fan of Van Halen, then wherever you see *Van Halen* here, just insert whatever is at the top of your list of stuff you really want to do in this lifetime—going to Hawaii, learning to paint, mastering the tango—whatever brings you true joy and leaves you grinning with anticipation every time you think about it. Okay?

Back in my school days, my room was covered in posters and clippings of Dave and Eddie and the band. I used to place the needle of my record player at the beginning of their record and set my stereo on a timer to wake up to them every morning. (Geez, what am I, eighty years old? And then we walked to the creek, beat our laundry on rocks, did some cave paintings, and invented fire.)

Anyway, the band split up before I ever had a chance to see them live. They've been feuding for more than twenty years, with rumors of reunions always dashed shortly after they arise, so when their reunion tour was finally announced, I told one of my friends, "We *must* go to the first concert. Those guys have such a hard time getting along, there probably won't be a second concert. There may not even be a second half of the first concert."

Now I really doubt that Dave is no longer an egomaniac or that Eddie has resolved all his issues, whatever they may be. Who knows how long they'll get along? If seeing Van Halen perform live (remember, insert your idea of utopia here) is on your list of things to do before you die, what are you waiting for? Remember, there may not be a second show. For them or for you.

• • •

Chapter 7

I'd Like to Speak to the Owner of This Body: Moving Forward and Taking Responsibility

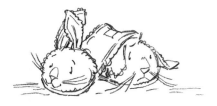

The Blame Game

My first reaction to my diagnosis was, like many folks, "Why me? What did I do to deserve this? Why am I being punished?" Apparently I wasn't the only one wondering this, as everyone around me seemed to have a causal theory for my illness, from toxins to viruses to genetics to sin.

I had two people from my church call me at different times. The kinder soul informed me that I was sick because I was doing God's work and the devil was attacking me, and the other informed me I was sick because I had some hidden sin in my life (and was being punished). Hmm. Can't be both now, can it?

I was surprised and hurt that people from my church were blaming me for my problems instead of bringing me casseroles. I was starting to feel like a leper from biblical times. Every time I left the house, I almost expected someone to run out in front of me yelling, "UNCLEAN! UNCLEAN!" How could they judge and abandon a fellow church member in her hour of greatest need?

Eventually, I realized they were just scared. If they could somehow blame it on me, they could convince themselves that it could never happen to them. That made it easier for me to forgive them. They probably didn't think they needed to be forgiven for anything, but I really needed to make peace with it.

Over time, I've become aware of just how much illness and suffering there are in the world. It seems like everybody has a sister or an aunt or a coworker with a serious illness or a deep personal tragedy. We don't get these things because we deserve them. If we did, there would be no book called *When Bad Things Happen to Good People;* instead there'd just be a pamphlet called *Isn't It Great That Only Mean People Get Sick?*

• • •

Don't Blame the Salad

Not taking the blame for my illness is healthy, but not taking responsibility is just asking for more problems. The fact is, our lifestyle choices, especially what we eat, have a great deal of influence over our health. The bad news: if you really want healing, it's up to you. The good news: if you really want healing, it's up to you. You're in the driver's seat. You can positively affect your well-being!

I had a friend who developed vasculitis and nearly died of kidney failure. The day before he landed in the hospital, he had a salad and was wearing a nicotine patch—while smoking. And what does he think was the last straw that triggered the illness? The salad. I'm not kidding. His life was saved by immune suppressants, and amazingly, the minute he left the hospital he went right back to smoking. He said to me, "Well, if this stuff is going to happen to me anyway, smoking isn't going to make a difference." Diagnosis is not blanket permission to self-destruct; it is a wake-up call telling us that how we were living isn't working for us and we need to change.

If you want to make unhealthy choices, no one can stop you; it's your body. But at least own up to the choice. Don't blame the salad.

• • •

How to Get and Stay Sick: A "To-Don't" List

Want to get sick and stay that way? Want to see if it's as fun as it looks? Follow these excellent suggestions, and you'll end up with something regrettable eventually.

- Eat crap and die (it's not just a pithy schoolyard comeback!). Not sure what crap is? Processed foods, preservatives, artificial colors and sweeteners, loads of sugar, and plenty of salt. You can find crap in every aisle of the grocery store, minus the produce section. Speaking of which: avoid all fruits and vegetables. They will screw up the eating-crap-and-dying process. Bonus: If you eat all that sugar, you can start a yeast farm on your tongue.

- Get six-pack abs: Pop open a can of soda for breakfast and enjoy the blood sugar roller coaster all day. Any kind will work. The aspartame in diet soda is damaging to your nervous system, and the high fructose corn syrup in regular soda can lead to diabetes. Also, drinking cola regularly may contribute to kidney problems. Now start doing those sixteen-ounce curls!

- Allergic to a food? Chow down on it! A little hair of the dog, that's what you need!

- Ask your dentist for plutonium fillings in your teeth. Can't get plutonium? Well, many dentists still make amalgam fillings with other toxic metals, including mercury, tin, and nickel.

- Don't brush or floss. Ever. If God had meant for us to brush our teeth, we would have plastic bristles on the ends of our hands, right? Let that bacteria build up in your gums so it can get into your bloodstream and go after your heart. Then blame your heart condition on bad luck.

- Drink lots of alcohol. Haven't you heard? Wine is good for you. So lots of wine must be *really* good for you, right? If you can't find wine with nitrates, then drink a twelve-pack of light beer a day. It's loaded with chemicals. More great news: alcohol depletes you of vitamins and minerals. So does caffeine, so chase your beer with a frappuccino.

- Take prescription drugs for fun. Everybody's doing it! If you're ever in pain, you'll need double the dose for it to work, but that's such a small price to pay for being able to numb yourself from all emotions. As a bonus, you'll probably be constipated.

- Take antibiotics for everything. This may eventually lead to getting an antibiotic-resistant infection. Think big!

- Move next door to a pesticide plant, or into an old house with lead pipes, lead paint, and asbestos. Drink the tap water from those rusty pipes without filtering or distilling it—that ruins the taste. If you can, find a place that also has a high-voltage power plant across the street and lots of overhead plane traffic. Add a crack house next door for excitement. Location, location, location!

- Sit around and do nothing. It's very Zen, you know. Be ultra-Zen: no fresh air, sunshine, other people, or exercise.

- Not good at doing nothing? Try martyrdom. Work all the time and put everyone else's needs and demands above your own. Others get sick from being lazy and irresponsible—you get to feel self-righteous.

- Don't do anything about that stress. Meditating is for weirdos.

- Hang out with the drama queens. Balanced people are so boring.

- Hang on to grudges and nurse them. Mmm, justifiable anger!

- Focus on everything that sucks. Stuck for ideas? Turn on the news.

- No laughing! This is serious! Do not have fun.

• • •

The Toxin Avenger

Toxins? When a naturopath first introduced me to the idea of toxins floating around in my body, it sounded like the kind of paranoid rant you'd hear on AM radio in the middle of the night from a guy wearing a tinfoil hat. But as I thought about it more, it made sense. There are a lot of substances that we know are toxic, like arsenic, lead, asbestos, hemlock, antifreeze. Hey, I watch *Forensic Files*.

Well, apparently there are lots of other substances that we expose ourselves to daily that are not healthy, like chemicals in cosmetics, deodorants, hair products, car exhaust, paint fumes, and formaldehyde in furniture and carpets, to name a few. Ick!

In *Never Be Sick Again*, Raymond Francis, MSc, theorizes that all diseases are caused by two things: nutritional deficiency and toxicity. Well, that's the best explanation I've heard for illness yet. If this is true, then it is almost entirely within my power to actually get well. Worth a shot.

"How do I detoxify?" I asked the naturopath.

"Coffee enemas!"

"What!? Let me get this straight. You want me to take a double latte and stick it *where*? Why would I do that? No way, no how, not happening!"

So there I was getting a coffee enema, singing "On the Commode Again."

It probably would have gone more smoothly if I had removed the little stir stick first.

Thankfully, after a little more research, I found out there are other means of detox. We have five eliminative organs (kidneys, colon, liver, lungs, and skin) and a lymphatic system. So you have some choices: water fasts and juices fasts (fasts should be supervised), massage, detox herbs and teas, poultices, bouncing on a good trampoline, and low-heat saunas (110° to 120°F).

Thankfully, I never really liked coffee in the first place, because I've never been able to look at it quite the same.

• • •

The War on War

Some doctors say those with autoimmune disorders have "hyperactive" immune systems. I don't know if our immune systems really are stronger than most people's. Maybe they're just confused, leaving the germs alone and going after the wrong "enemies," like vital organs. How did my immune system become my "frenemy"?

In his syndicated column *To Your Good Health*, Dr. Paul G. Donahue describes *autoimmunity* as the immune system producing "a slew of antibodies—immune system grenades—and [tossing] them at many organs."

Grenades. Yeah, that's a good metaphor. It feels like war. Specifically, it feels like the "war on terror," with an elusive enemy we don't really understand, who lives among us and is unpredictable. When we bomb the enemy (with drugs), we take a lot of collateral damage (horrible side effects), and while we're fighting the enemy in one place, we're left vulnerable elsewhere (a squashed immune system). In the end, all we can hope for is to contain the terror as much as possible and hope we don't run out of resources.

Sadly, I don't think a war on terror can be won. The best we can hope for in a war situation is a tenuous peace, which is the same we hope for with autoimmune disease: a long, deep, or even permanent remission.

We are not alone. Anyone who struggles with addiction, yo-yo dieting, OCD, hoarding, or gambling knows that you can't just win the war and be done with it. Once something like that has a foothold in your life, it is always near, ready to infiltrate and take over. We have to keep vigilant without letting the problem take over our minds, however. According to the World Health Organization, health is defined as "a state of complete physical, mental and social well-being, not merely the absence of disease or infirmity."

To achieve "world peace" in our bodies, we have to use not just the weapons that tear down disease (drugs, chemo, surgery) but also the tools that build up health (alternative medicine, spirituality, nutrition, exercise, rest, love). We also need to find out what was making the enemy so mad in the first place and stop doing it (e.g., stop eating garbage). Maybe then we have a chance at real, lasting peace.

• • •

Illness as Metaphor

As a songwriter, I'm always looking beneath the surface of things for deeper meanings. I spend so much time reading between the lines that I can't get through a dinner menu without finding a subtext. So, of course, I often find myself thinking about what it means to have a chronic illness, or any illness. Is it a metaphor? What does it represent? Why is it here? Why this particular illness? What can I learn from it? What is it trying to tell me? What does it *mean?* (And how can I get rid of it?!)

So when I met a woman who called herself a medical hypnotist, I started a conversation. She casually mentioned, as if it were common knowledge, "Oh, yes. All illness starts at an energetic level. By the time it manifests itself physically, it is a metaphor." Holy cow! I knew it, I knew it, I knew it!

Before I was ill, Jesse, one of my coworkers, lost a dear friend. His friend had recovered from her cancer, only to die of pneumonia. Jesse was so angry with his friend's doctors that his anger literally consumed him, and within a year he died of a cancerous tumor wrapped around his heart. It certainly doesn't take a perceptive songwriter to figure out that metaphor. Had they been able to remove his tumor, I have the sneaking suspicion that he would have grown another one somewhere else, because he was still angry, sad, and unresolved. It's like dealing with weeds. You can mow them, cut them, and pull them up, but if you don't get rid of the roots and the seeds, they'll just come right back.

So what does *my* illness mean? If autoimmune disease occurs when your immune system can't tell "self" from "nonself," perhaps the metaphor was that I had become something I wasn't. I had created a life that was so opposed to my authentic self that maybe my immune system didn't recognize me anymore. I don't know to what degree my emotional state contributes to illness, but being that close to death was the wake-up call I needed to change my situation. This is the greatest gift this illness has given me—permission to be who I really am.

● ● ●

And the Broom She Rode In On: Making a Clean Sweep

In the end, it is important to remember that we cannot become what we need to be by remaining what we are.

—Max DePree

I'm just fascinated by TV shows like *Clean Sweep* and *Clean House*. Folks write in to the show asking for help, and if you're one of the lucky families to be chosen, the team shows up, takes all the junk out of your house, puts it on the lawn, and makes you sort it into three piles: keep, toss, or sell. Then they have a big yard sale, donate the leftovers to charity, redecorate and organize, and have a big "reveal" at the end.

Most of us never do this in our own houses because, without some outside help, the task is overwhelming. (And without a big truck outside that says TV CREW, it's hard to explain to your neighbors why everything you own is on the lawn being sorted out onto various tarps.) Further, sometimes we really need some help convincing ourselves to let go of things that just aren't working for us anymore.

The year I first fell ill, nothing in my life was working. As I'm sure I've mentioned by now, I hated my job, I was a very involved member of a less-than-compassionate church, and I lived in a dumpy trailer park. Even my cat was miserable—he had fleas I couldn't seem to get rid of and a flea allergy that made his fur fall out. My whole life needed a clean sweep. In this way, the illness was a blessing.

It's so much easier to leave a job you hate, a town that just doesn't seem to work for you, and an uninhabitable home when you've been forced out by an illness.

I "redesigned" my life—this time on purpose, not by default. I got a small apartment, which I loved; went back to teaching guitar, which I loved; and was now living in my hometown, which I loved. I spent a lot of time writing, which I love; joined a bicycle club; and made friends through making music. Everything in my life was now there on purpose, and all the old clutter that was holding me down was gone. My cat even recovered from his flea problem and became his old happy, playful self.

Sometimes when I'm watching these "clean-up" shows, I think to myself, "What's going to keep these people from just cluttering the house back up?" If they never deal with the behaviors that got them to that point (such as compulsive shopping, hoarding, or bad housekeeping habits), then it's just a matter of time before they're calling the show back and saying, "Can you come back and clean our house again?"

Eventually, this is what happened to me. I fell back into measuring my self-worth the way our society does, by how much money you make and how well known you are. I started to stress out about getting ahead instead of just allowing myself to be happy doing what I love. Then I invited the crazy people back into my life—people who suck the life out of you. I quit paying attention to what I ate, stopped taking care of myself, and put everything else above that priority. Maybe I didn't feel I deserved all that love I was giving myself. In the end, I really messed up my "house" again, and nine years after I was first diagnosed with lupus, I had a pair of strokes. With a great deal of help from a "clean sweep" team of friends and health practitioners, I recovered completely and began doing a superb job caring for myself again.

After a couple years of good health, I got all swept up in "making something of myself" again. I decided (yet again) that everything else in the world was more important than taking good care of myself. My boyfriend (now husband) kept telling me, "If you keep this up, you're going to end up in the hospital again." Yeah, yeah. Lo and behold, four years after the strokes, I did indeed end up in the hospital again. (Who could have seen that coming? I mean besides everybody.)

Times when we are beaten down are usually our most teachable moments. In twelve-step programs they call this "hitting a bottom"—where you're so beat up by your own behavior you're actually ready to try something new. It's the tipping point where your coping mechanisms (drinking, hoarding, numbing out with work or food) are causing more pain than they are relieving. At that moment, we are ready to throw those self-destructive habits on the "toss" pile—even though it feels like getting rid of your favorite cushy (nasty, stinky, dirty) chair.

Sometimes people get real with the host of *Clean House* and talk about what caused their lives to spiral out of control or admit to the habits that are contributing to their predicament. Whenever I see a family member take responsibility and make a plan to develop new habits, I feel some hope that maybe the house will stay clean.

We all love a Cinderella story—it makes for great TV: horribly messy house, team comes in and rescues the family from their own mess, paints everything, does the "big reveal," and leaves. But what about the "happily ever after"? What happens when the cameras go away?

An intervention is a beautiful act of giving, but we can't keep tearing our lives apart and then expect those around us to keep fixing it for us. At some point, they're either going to get disgusted or run out of resources and leave us to our own devices. They have their own lives to run. We have to find ways to get our needs met without letting it become a crisis. It's so much easier to keep a house clean than it is to demolish and rebuild it.

• • •

Patient, Heal Thyself

Take your life in your own hands and what happens? A terrible thing: no one to blame.

—Erica Jong

Lupus is pretty much a DIY (do it yourself) illness. If you're struggling with lupus—or any serious or chronic illness—you've probably figured this out by now. Diseases don't always follow a predictable path, so keeping your own health history is a great way to start to take the wheel and be in charge of your own recovery, rather than just be at the mercy of the disease's symptoms and the drug side effects. (I don't know about you, but I can't afford to leave my well-being in the hands of a medical person I spend six minutes with every three months, even if he's nice.)

My health history, which I keep up-to-date when I'm in a crisis/recovery, includes:

> **Pill list.** This includes everything I'm taking, how many milligrams, how many times a day, including any over the counter drugs (aspirin, ibuprofen, etc.), supplements, and vitamins. Don't look at this every day (unless you need it

to keep track of what to take; I use a plastic slotted pill organizer from the drug store for that). Update this whenever something changes, including reduction of dosage. Especially for heavy drugs, such as prednisone. Every time I cut back on prednisone, I felt like I was going into a relapse when, in fact, I was usually just going through prednisone withdrawal. Since I was keeping a journal, I noticed that after I cut back on prednisone, I would feel lousy for a few days, then the feelings passed. Otherwise, I might have panicked after one day and gone to the doctor to jack the prednisone back up. This list is also important for the doctor, who can check it for potential drug interactions.

List of diagnoses. Update this if you get a new one. Don't look at it every day. This is something to write down so you don't *have* to think about it. Include date of diagnosis and treatment given.

List of allergies, especially drug allergies. Update it if something new develops. Again, don't look at it every day. It's just something to have on hand for the doctor/hospital so they don't accidentally kill you with antibiotics or iodine tests.

List of doctors, hospitals you've been admitted to, and other health practitioners. Don't forget people like your acupuncturist and your dentist, and include phone numbers and addresses for all of them. Update it whenever you have a new doctor or other health practitioner.

List of surgeries. Include dates, physician names, and the hospitals where the surgeries were performed. Update when needed, but don't look at this unless you need to fill out a form requesting this info.

Copies of lab results. Request these from the lab when you go, or pay your doctor later for copies. By law, you are allowed copies, though there may be a small fee.

Photo. A picture of yourself healthy and happy. This is the goal. Put it on the front cover, where you will see it every day.

Daily status log. This is the section you use daily. Just leave it open to the latest page and jot down something quick in the morning about whatever you're monitoring and trying to improve. Some entries may be for things that happened the day before. Things to include:

- Weight. This is important because unexplained weight loss is a symptom of active disease. Also, unusual weight gain can signal kidney problems (water retention), or just be a side effect of prednisone (again, water retention).

- Blood pressure, if this is an issue for you. Do not rely on the freestanding machines at drugstores, which are frequently inaccurate because they haven't been calibrated. You can purchase a motorized battery-operated blood pressure monitor at any major drugstore. (Don't try to use a manual one to check your own blood pressure. Trust me on that.)

- Pain level. (On a scale of 0 to 10, 0 = pain free and 10 = unbearable.)

- Temperature. Take it *before* drinking anything cold or hot, and do not take it right after a hot or cold shower or after exercising. All those things will give you abnormal readings. I take mine as soon as I get up every day.

- Energy level. (On a scale of 0 to 10, 0 = exhausted and 10 = positively peppy.)

- Any current symptoms.

- Medical treatments received that day (tests, transfusion, physical therapy, dental work, etc.).

- Alternative treatments received that day (acupuncture, massage, chelation, chiropractic, etc.).

- Self-care for the day (walking, qigong, other exercise; psychotherapy/support group, journaling).

- Fun/joyous activities that day (outings, get-togethers, etc.).

The graph. This is the final piece, and do look at this one regularly. This is my little invention to motivate myself by tracking progress. You can create more than one graph, but I like to keep it all on one page. (You can see an example on my Web site, www.thesingingpatient.com.) I got a piece of graph paper and put markers for my weight, pain level, temperature, energy level along the left side, and the dates along the bottom. Along the top of the page, I put a little asterisk on days I did something fun and/or had alternative treatments. I use different colored pens to mark points on the graph for each thing I track.

Some things you want to go up (energy, maybe weight) and others down (pain, maybe weight). You can also add any lab test numbers and graph them.

Why do I add fun activities to the chart? Fun activities boost your health. Remember, happiness is good for you and a positive event such as a fun gathering with family or friends can positively affect you for thirty-six hours. I purposely schedule regular, fun activities.

It's important to stay ability-focused and celebrate what we are able to do instead of concentrating on what we can't do. This puts us back in control and keeps us continuously motivated to stretch ourselves to do more and regain more of our former abilities. For me, the chart is a very useful tool in keeping this focus.

Once I'm feeling fine, I generally stop doing the journal and just put it away in a file. I start a new one when/if everything goes downhill again. My second and third journals I did on a computer rather than in a spiral notebook. I am seeking a balance between being responsible about this whole thing (regular blood tests and doctor visits, self-care, eating well, exercise) and just living my life fully, as free of disease as possible, in body as well as mind.

• • •

Chapter 8

The Early Bird Can Have the Worm: Pacing Yourself

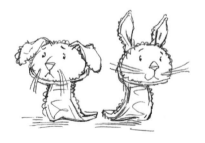

The Stress Test

We little realize the number of human diseases that are begun
or affected by worry.
—Walter Clement Alvarez, MD

Stress—it's enough to make anyone sick! In my case, because I was sick, I was stressed out because I couldn't work, I couldn't keep up with the household chores, and I had a pile of medical bills. Then I found out that stress aggravates my condition, and now I was stressed out about the stress. Stress is the worst thing for autoimmunity, and stressing about autoimmunity is the strangest irony I can think of. Except maybe stressing about stress.

Sometimes I wish I could just have a beer (not an option) or go for a jog to blow off some steam (not an option). Or drink a ton of coffee and just power through the stress (not an option). Since indulging in any of these things would actually cause more problems for me than they would solve, I'm forced to figure out some other way to deal with stress—hopefully in a healthy manner. However, like everything else that seems to be a limitation, maybe it's really an opportunity to learn some new skills.

It became apparent that I needed to deal with the root of the problem. The fact is, most of my stress is created between my ears. Much of it is not what happens, but what I think about it and how I react to it. I tried taking an anti-anxiety medication, but eventually I developed a tolerance to it, so it didn't work anymore. Plus, it was wiping out my short-term memory. While this is great for enjoying the same TV shows over and over, it's not so great for being a functional human being.

I tried to learn to meditate. But that required me to not think and, well, I'm kind of addicted to thinking. It's my last remaining vice. I mean, for heaven's sake, I gave up pizza and diet soda! Just how good a human do I have to be? Why am I arguing with a blank page?

If there's a particular person, place or thing that's stressing me out, I can try to limit my exposure. But I often find I'm upset or even obsessing about things I can't control. If I can't do anything about it, there's no point in worrying about it. And if I can do something about it, there's still no point in worrying—just make a plan and start doing. Sometimes the Serenity Prayer helps with this: God (or universe), grant me the serenity to accept the things I cannot change, the courage to change the things I can, and the wisdom to know the difference. (And give it to me right now!)

I'm still learning how to deal with stress. For now, when I just want to take my mind off things, I go for a walk, talk with a friend, do something fun or creative, have a good laugh, or just take some long, deep breaths. Because you gotta decompress— I can't stress that enough.

• • •

Energy Policy

A well-spent day brings happy sleep.
—**Leonardo da Vinci**

The fact is, when you're in the middle of fighting off an active disease, you have to make hard choices every day about how to spend your limited energy.

At one point, while I was recovering from a bad flare-up, one of my friends suggested we go shopping and have dinner, and maybe earlier that day we could go do something else. I had to explain—both to her and myself—that at that point I could do only one big thing a day. If I scheduled two events, I might survive them both, but there won't be enough of me left to enjoy the second one, and it would ruin me for the next day.

If I paced myself and did only one big thing a day, I could very well end up doing thirty really neat things in a month. Well, maybe only twenty-six, because sometimes my one big thing is laundry. Still, twenty-six neat things a month—barbecues with friends, going to the arcade, doing a gig—is pretty great. But if I don't pace myself when I'm not well, I can end up wasting a lot of time flat on my back in bed watching reruns, staring out the window, and popping pills to kill the pain.

When I'm recovering, I can either go to the arcade, or I can cook dinner. I can either wash and blow-dry my hair, or I can go to the grocery store. (I'll probably never make it to the grocery store with freshly styled hair.) I can either putter around in the garden, or I can go to the gym.

The good part about knowing that you have limited resources is (hopefully) you don't squander those resources on stupid stuff. It's an opportunity to make more deliberate choices about how and with whom you spend your time—a skill that is equally useful when you're well.

• • •

Fibromyalgia: The Other F Word

During and even between my three episodes of active illness, I've had one nearly constant companion: fibromyalgia. After the big scares have all passed—my kidneys are no longer failing, I've recovered from the stroke, the neuropathy has subsided, etc.— the pain has almost always still been there.

I find that the fibro pain doesn't seem to register with my doctors, because it's not measurable on a blood test or an X-ray. All this time I've been pretty much on my own in dealing with the fibro. I'm not the only one. People all over the world are muttering "the other *F* word" under their breath every day.

I tried so many things to remedy the fatigue, the tenderness in my arms, the brain fog and irritability, and the tightness and pain in my upper back that keep me awake at night: chiropractic, stretching, ignoring and denying, popping lots of ibuprofen, massage, capsaicin patches, Icy Hot, a TENS unit, a heating pad, gentle exercise, not-so-gentle exercise, meditation, journaling, and staying educated. For me, I'd say the least-effective technique has been ignoring and denying, though for some reason I hung on to that tactic the longest.

The most effective for me? Chinese acupuncture, qigong, detox, stress management, rest, diet change (getting rid of junk food and diet soda), facing my feelings, and having fun. Faith, hope, and joy are the kinds of emotions that cause healthy chemical changes in the body. How you feel emotionally affects how you feel physically.

I have been free from fibromyalgia pain for months (praise the Lord and knock on wood!), so for now, there's only one *F* word in my life—the naughty one. And since I'm not in pain, I seem to need to mutter that one a little less often, too.

• • •

How Not to Be Completely Exhausted

Where do you dredge for energy when you are seriously ill? I've tried many things over the years of having autoimmune diseases follow me around and sit on me like a hippo. Really, the following tips apply to anyone, even healthy people:

1. Know when to quit. As the Russian proverb goes, "If you feel an urge to work, take a nap, and it will pass."

2. Take as little painkiller as is effective. If I can take one-quarter or one-half of a narcotic pill for pain, I'll be less groggy than if I had taken a whole tablet. And less constipated. Do take enough to get the pain under control, though; otherwise you'll ultimately end up taking even more. If you've had a procedure, like a wisdom tooth extraction, take the pills as prescribed; do not wait until the pain inevitably kicks in. Don't ask me how I know.

3. Drink less caffeine. Yes, you're more tired for the first few days, but caffeine makes your energy fluctuate big time and then keeps you awake. I've given up on eliminating

it completely, but I just have one glass of green tea when I get up, and that's it. I've seen enough really bad late-night TV. (Oh great! Another episode of "paid programming.")

4. Consume less sugar. Sugar also sends your energy all over the place. I have come to like Stevia (an acquired taste), a natural plant derivative with no calories. I was on a candida (antiyeast–no carb) diet for one and a half years, and I felt amazing. I was seduced by a birthday cake and fell off the wagon, but I still don't indulge like I once did.

5. Learn to meditate, if only for five minutes a day. Thinking uses energy, and allowing your brain to "spin" is like leaving your car idling. Meditation quiets the mind.

6. Find a way to restore your chi (life force/energy). Acupuncture has been really effective for me—even though I can't stand needles. Acupuncture needles are much smaller than most needles you encounter at the phlebotomist. Sometimes I don't feel the acupuncture needles at all. Should you decide to give acupuncture a try, ask around first for a good practitioner. (I always talk to another patient when I am looking for a health care provider of any kind. Getting a referral has seriously cut back on my number of unpleasant experiences.) If you can't get a personal recommendation, go online and search for someone who does Five Element acupuncture, or look up the Accreditation Commission for Acupuncture and Oriental Medicine for a practitioner in your area.

Sometimes acupuncturists also treat with herbs, which can be an indication of deeper training. Word to the wise: there is a big difference between a licensed acupuncturist, who has had years of training, and an MD who happens to offer acupuncture. MDs can get licensed in acupuncture with as little as one weekend's worth of training. I've also found qigong to be so effective for restoring my energy that if I practice it when I get up, I don't even need caffeine that day.

7. Detox. We have five organs that eliminate toxins from the body—kidneys, colon, liver, lungs, and skin—plus the lymphatic system. Of the many detox methods out there, I have personally tried massage, lymphatic massage, a rebounder (a mini-trampoline), coffee enemas (!), juice fasting, chelation therapy (removes heavy metals from the system via IV treatment or pills), low-heat sauna, baths, various herbs, and deep breathing. I have yet to try herbal wraps or poultices, but some people swear by them. Unless you live somewhere so remote that you can't even get a copy of this book, you need to detox.

8. Exercise. The trick is to exercise enough to get your heart rate up but not work so hard that you set yourself back (see number 1). If the only exercise you've had in years is a sixteen-ounce curl, don't run to the gym and start doing squat thrusts. It's going to take a while to work your way back up to your former high school glory. Let's say your goal is to spend sixty minutes on the

treadmill six days a week. If even twenty minutes is too much, start with ten or even five and increase the duration over time. After I had a stroke, I started even smaller: I stood in the pool, holding on to the side, and kicked for a few minutes. When I was strong enough, I walked to the stop sign and back. The goal is progress, starting from where you are right now. You are your own yardstick against which to measure your progress.

9. Reduce inflammation. Some doctors recommend one tablespoon of pure, mercury-free fish or flax oil daily, such as Barlean's. Turmeric and curcumin are also said to reduce inflammation. An anti-inflammatory diet would consist mostly of plant foods, little salt or sugar, and little or no animal products (such as meat and dairy).

10. Take a daily multivitamin. Don't skimp. Get a good one derived from actual food (that is, naturally occurring ingredients) rather than one synthesized from petrochemicals. Unfortunately, many vitamins on the market are coated with sugar or held together with artificial chemical binders. At one time I was taking some vitamin B complex because I was tired, and the vitamin tablet made me even more tired! I later learned that the cheaper, chemically synthesized vitamin B can cause that effect. (*Note:* Be sure to mention any supplements or herbs you are taking to your doctor to avoid drug interactions.) No more cheap vitamins—yabba dabba doo!

11. Drink water. The human body is 55 to 60 percent water. Dehydration makes you tired. Filter or distill water at home to get rid of those pharmaceuticals floating around in many municipal water supplies.

That's all I can think of for now. It's time to follow suggestion number 1—know when to quit!

• • •

Some See My Glass as Half Full. I Say, "Glass? What Glass?"

Shortly after my third bout of illness, there I was again, running myself into the ground. You know, trying to live at the pace everyone else does even though I had active disease and had just had a terrible relapse eight months before. Through sheer willpower, I planned my wedding and went on numerous trips, most business, a few pleasure.

One of those pleasure trips was to a weeklong guitar retreat (grown-up "guitar camp") with my newlywed husband. We both play guitar—in fact, that's how we met—so it was kind of an extension of our honeymoon. I love guitar camp, but it is exhausting. Classes start at 9:00 a.m. and go all day, and then everyone stays up until 2:00 or 3:00 a.m. jamming and swapping songs. I was having a blast, but I was depleting myself.

The universe was looking out for me, however. I met this guy the last night of camp, and it turned out that he was an MD *and* a Chinese medicine practitioner. He ended up basically giving me a long free consult. After looking at my tongue (this is normal for Chinese practitioners), asking me a bunch of questions, and hearing my medical history, Dr. Sal gave me the wag of the finger. He bluntly asked me if I wanted to live longer than just a couple more years. If so, I was going to have to make some big changes. It was a major wake-up call.

The big lesson was to stop using up all my chi (life force, energy). Anyone who has a chronic illness understands this conundrum—as soon as you feel the least bit good, you get so excited that you run out and do everything you've wanted to do but haven't been able to because you were too tired before. Then you deplete yourself and wind up in bed for several days. It reminds me of the saying "money burns a hole in his pocket" and the mentality that describes.

Dr. Sal explained it to me in just such a metaphor: A rich man was asked how he stayed rich. He said his wealth was like a full glass that dripped over the sides. He lived off the extra water dripping over the rim, never drinking from the actual glass. In other words, you never dip into the principal; you just live off the dividends and interest. I had to stop drinking from the glass and let it fill up, instead of using every bit of energy I had and leaving nothing for my body to repair and balance itself with.

Some days I just had to accept that I wasn't going to get much done on the old to-do list. I had to "fill up my glass." Through practicing qigong, I now have a way to actively fill the glass rather than just waiting for it to fill itself.

Some see the glass as half empty. Some see it as half full. I see it being slowly filled up.

• • •

The Qigong Show

Qigong is a Chinese healing art that was developed for the purpose of cultivating qi (life force, or chi) in pursuit of immortality. Qigong is similar to tai chi in that it is a series of slow, gentle physical movements. After having numerous practitioners and books suggest I try qigong, I finally learned a set of five gentle exercises that I now practice regularly. I'm not hoping to achieve immortality—just hoping to be full of life while I'm here on the planet.

It really is remarkable how much more energy and focus I have on the days I do qigong versus the days I do not. The simple routine I have learned only takes me about ten minutes, which makes you wonder why I wouldn't do it every day—or even twice a day. Perhaps it's my ego. There's nothing in qigong to appeal to my macho side. It's extremely *not* flashy. The moves have names like Putting a Lid on a Pot, Ball Holding, and the Wind Sways the Lotus Leaves. (I can hear it now: "Stand back, buddy, or I'll sway the wind through your leaves!") Contrary to something like karate, there is no "boot to the head" in qigong. Maybe "woman slowly lifts boot and places it gently on own head."

There's also nothing in qigong that leads directly to achieving a big, impressive goal. When I get bored by other exercise—such as walking, bike riding, or swimming—I can fantasize about running the Rocky steps in Philadelphia, crossing a finish line, or swimming in a triathlon. When I do qigong, it's so I can have enough energy to go grocery shopping or mop the floor. Some fantasy. And there's certainly no "Hey y'all, check this out!" when it comes to doing qigong. From a spectator standpoint, watching someone do qigong is less interesting than watching paint dry. (Really attractive paint, of course.)

Back in the 1970s, it was the mission of *The Gong Show* to find the worst in entertainment and put it on TV. Three celebrity judges stood by, mallet in hand, waiting for a chance to gong the acts off the stage. I'm betting a qigong act would have received a gong from all three judges.

Ultimately, I practice qigong not so I can show it off to others or to knock someone's block off, but to heal my body and cultivate my life force. I don't know how or why it makes me feel better, but it does. Like so many other things I have done to regain my health, I can't really afford to care if the whole world is standing there in front of a gong with a mallet, telling me what I'm doing is weird or boring. Anyway, what's so wrong with being weird? Millions of people loved Tiny Tim.

Anyone can follow the herd; it takes courage to be true to yourself. You're invited to tune in every day around noon to *The*

Qigong Show, where I'll be putting lids on pots and maybe even placing a boot gently on my head. Leave your mallet at home.

• • •

Chapter 9

Mirror, Mirror, on the Wall, Who's the . . . Oh, Never Mind: Beauty

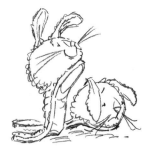

Wigging Out

I've lost my hair three times over the years, due to disease as well as treatments. My hair is extremely thick when it's healthy, so the thinning doesn't show right away. I hide the problem for as long as I can, restyling it and wearing hats, but eventually, I just have to cut off what straggly hair is left and start over. I'd love to just shave my head, but with a bald head, an eighty-two-pound body, and a puffed-up, moon-pie prednisone face . . . I'd look like a lollipop. Add my swollen feet, and I'd look like a Q-Tip.

It was during my second autoimmune episode that I bought a wig. Nice human-hair wigs cost hundreds of dollars, and that was not in my budget, so I got a cheap $40 nylon wig. I figured everyone would know it was fake hair, but the first day I wore it out, a clerk in a store commented on my great haircut! She made my day.

Interestingly, the wig became a barometer for how comfortable I was with a person. When I was at a friend's house, I often found myself taking the wig off, because I felt like he accepted me and didn't judge me on how good or bad I looked. A couple of times I left it in a chair and scared the heck out of him—he thought a small animal had snuck into the house. I guess I'm lucky his dog didn't get a hold of it.

One chilly day in January, a bunch of us were at a folk festival. I had performed already—my first time playing guitar in public since the strokes. I hadn't fully regained my guitar-playing abilities, and I could only play a few songs. I had just stopped using a cane to walk, and my balance wasn't good. I really had no business being out and about that particular day, but it made me so happy to be among friends.

Some of us were standing around backstage toward the end of the night, and my friend and I were cutting up. I laughed so hard that I lost my balance and fell over—and my wig fell off! The sad part was that I was still too weak to get up off the ground by myself.

Thankfully I was among people who cared about me—they showed the proper amount of concern and helped peel me off the ground, and then we all had a good laugh about how I literally "laughed my head off." I learned that those friends didn't judge me for wearing a wig, or for looking silly. I suppose it's also a lesson in the importance of using bobby pins.

I've always been able to taper off the prednisone completely after about a year on it, so eventually my hair comes back, and when it finally does, it's dark and curly. (Between the wild weight fluctuations, the prednisone face, and the change in hair, I've often said I missed my window of opportunity to commit crimes. No one could have identified me.) Right now I have a full head of my own hair again.

Somewhere I still have my wig in a box. I'm a little superstitious about it now. When I gave away my expensive prescription panty hose (the kind used to reduce swelling/water retention in your legs due to kidney problems), I ended up needing them a few months later. While I was annoyed that I had to repurchase the hose, I was more upset that my kidneys were failing again. Some part of me feels that if I keep my wig, I'll never need it again. I can find lots of other ways to laugh my head off.

• • •

Hair's the Problem: Eighteen Tips for Better Hair

Regardless of how you feel physically, I don't see anything wrong with wanting to look good. Whenever I'm seriously ill, it seems like all any doctor ever cares about is saving my kidneys. Kidneys, schmidneys! What about my hair? Did people *ooh* and *aah* over Marilyn Monroe's kidneys? Or remark on Jennifer Aniston's beautiful pancreas?

More than once I've had to choose between saving my kidneys and keeping my hair. The kidneys always win, but not without some hesitation on my part. I do the chemo, or take the drugs, or both, and find myself pulling blobs of hair the size of small rodents from the shower drain. It's incredibly depressing, but I never completely give up on my hair.

Here are a few things I've done to improve my hair situation during my medications-versus-hair dilemmas. Some of these may work for you:

1. Use leave-in conditioner. You can buy a conditioner that you just spray onto wet hair before putting a comb

through it. It helps the comb run smoothly through your hair without getting snagged, which reduces a lot of damage. You can also buy a detangler, which you use in the shower. It works just as well. Or you can get a serum made of natural oils that you apply to wet hair after the shower. Use this sparingly, so your hair doesn't get greasy.

2. Air- or towel-dry your hair before blow-drying to cut down on damage. Use the blow dryer sparingly and leave a little moisture in your hair.

3. Do not shampoo every day, especially if your hair is medium to long. I read somewhere that long-haired Hollywood stars are advised by "hair experts" to wash their tresses only two or three times a month. ("I'm sorry, I can't go out with you Friday night. I have to stay home and wash my—oh, um—socks.")

4. Use a deep conditioner once a week, like hot oil or three-minute deep conditioners.

5. Get regular haircuts to remove the dead ends. Dead, dry split ends do not make your hair look longer, just drier and unhealthy.

6. Use control paste (a dab smaller than a dime) to make the ends less frizzy. Rub it between your palms, and then work it into your hair, starting from the ends. If you get too much of it near the roots, it makes your hair look greasy and unwashed. (That's control paste, not glue. Elmer's glue is good for styling your hair into a mohawk.)

7. Use "shine" hair gloss or jojoba oil. Again, a dab'll do ya; work it in from the ends. This returns the shine your hair loses when you're full of drugs and not metabolizing nutrients normally or even when your hair is damaged from being overprocessed.

8. Use curlers (*not* hot curlers, but the kind you just put in when your hair is damp and leave in until it's dry) for special occasions to make your hair look fuller.

9. Use natural products as much as you can. I use healthy shampoo and conditioner, such as those made by Burt's Bees, that have no perfumes or sodium laurel sulfate, an unnecessarily harsh cleaner found in most shampoos.

10. Install a water purifier in your shower. A purifier is better than a filter alone—it removes more stuff than just chlorine and lead. Since I've had mine installed, my hair is softer, and it's not being exposed to chlorine and other chemicals every time I shower. I bought my purifier online, and it took me thirty seconds to install.

11. Get a *good* swim cap (like a Speedo racing cap) if you swim in a chlorinated pool. Swimming is good for you; chlorine is not. Anyone remember green hair from childhood summers in the pool?

12. Get a wig. If you've lost so much hair that you can see your scalp, or you have curly hair growing in under your straight hair and it's making the hair stick straight up

(been there, done that!), get yourself a wig. Unfortunately, as far as I know, Locks of Love (the organization that supplies free wigs of donated human hair) deals only with cancer patients. Some health care plans may cover at least part of the cost of a wig, but only if your doctor prescribes it as a "necessary cranial prosthesis" (I am not making this up). I was not in such a position, so I went shopping with my most princessy adult friend and got myself that nice $40 discount synthetic wig.

13. Wear hats and hairpieces. One of my friends who has thin hair—she's not ill; she was just born with thin hair—had an especially cute 'do one day. I complimented her on it, and she told me it was a hairpiece she bought at the dollar store! For a dollar! I've also seen long and short ponytails at the drugstore for quite reasonable prices. This is only for special occasions, especially if the hairpiece is heavy and pulls on your natural hair.

14. Color it. Some folks will tell you shouldn't be exposing yourself to more chemicals while you're sick (what do you think all those drugs are?). Maybe they're right, but looking in the mirror and hating my hair every day isn't good for me either. The way I feel emotionally affects the way I feel physically, and not wanting to leave the house because I feel unattractive is also bad for my mental health. Use low- or no-ammonia hair color. (FYI: If you color your hair yourself, do it outside the house. That stuff stinks!) *Note:* Sometimes certain drugs and even supplements can keep your hair from absorbing the dye. For a more natural solution, use henna.

15. Fix it from the inside. The health of our hair and skin (and nails) and our appearance in general is a reflection of our inner health. The best treatment for our hair is to improve our health. One baby step that directly improves hair: take flaxseed/flaxseed oil. It makes your hair grow faster and gives it shine. (And it helps keep you "regular"! Wahoo!) A quality multivitamin is also a good idea.

16. Do *not* get hair extensions or weaves, unless you have permanent hair loss. In the end, getting extensions does a lot of damage to your real hair, so eventually you have to cut it even shorter.

17. Use only a wide-tooth comb to detangle wet hair. Use a round brush to style when you blow-dry hair for fullness.

18. Massage your scalp regularly to stimulate circulation and hair growth.

For those of us with hair loss due to prednisone use, have faith: the hair will usually grow back (assuming you eventually get off the prednisone). Hair regrowth is not a given if you have the cutaneous (skin) form of lupus, genetic baldness, or alopecia. But if your hair loss is caused by any other illness or is a drug side effect, it should grow back.

Hair's to you!

• • •

Clothes Do Not Make the Man (or Woman)

Clothes make the man
Machines make the clothes
Man makes machines
Clothes make the man
—"Clothes Make the Man," Gregory Fleeman

I cleaned out my closet recently so I could see my useful clothes instead of having that staring-at-the-open-fridge kind of experience where you can't find the good stuff for all the clutter. Then, shortly after the purge, an interesting thing happened. Not one but *two* people gave me their castoff clothing, which was very nice stuff.

One person gave me her sweaters because they were too heavy for South Carolina (and I really need sweaters in New Jersey), and another, who had just lost a lot of weight, gave me her "fat" clothes.

This happened to me before, ten or so years ago, when I got six giant Hefty bags of clothes from two different friends who had both, in this case, gained weight and gave me their "skinny" clothes. (Interestingly, those "skinny" clothes were the same size as the "fat" clothes I just received.)

I've weighed everywhere from 82 to 150 pounds with this illness. When I'm ill, I lose muscle and appetite, and when I'm on the drugs, I retain a lot of water and gain as much as ten pounds a week. I fluctuate more than a high school wrestler wearing a plastic suit in a sauna. So I pretty much just wear T-shirts and pants with either drawstrings or elastic waists, or breezy pullover dresses. Otherwise, I would have to buy new clothes every two weeks. Also, clothes without zippers and buttons are easy to put on when your hands aren't working quite right. Choosing these types of clothes may not make me a fashion plate, but it means I can retain some dignity and independence by being able to dress myself.

I am not defined by my fat clothes, or my skinny clothes, or my ability or lack thereof to fit into them!

• • •

I'm Not Ready for My Close-up, Mr. DeMille

Let us not forget that a man can never get away from himself.
—Johann Wolfgang von Goethe

During one of my hospital stays, one of my girliest friends brought me a pile of fashion magazines. It was the most well-intended gesture, but it was so depressing to look at beautiful women at a time when I couldn't have felt less attractive. Even the always-entertaining "Guess whose cellulite-ridden legs these are?" photos didn't cheer me up.

During this, my decidedly least-sexy summer, my feet were too swollen to wear shoes. I had to wear slippers everywhere—the drug store, the doctor, the restaurant. What a fashion statement. (Well, at least I didn't have to worry about matching my socks.) My housemates had a big dog, and he liked to grab the slippers and run off with them—and he didn't always wait for me to take them off.

It's not just that I could wear only slippers; I couldn't find any *normal* slippers. The only ones I could find were huge pillowlike slippers with animal faces on them. They're so puffy, you have to walk upstairs sideways in them. And they're hot. Who needs this much cushion around the sides of their feet? It was like wearing giant sponges—with eyes. *Glamour* magazine missed a lot of opportunities to put me on their "don't" page that summer. The *National Enquirer* missed three entire months of "bigfoot" sightings.

My ankles were puffy, too—so swollen, in fact, that I couldn't wear jeans. I put a pair on one morning, and by afternoon my ankles were so swollen that I had to cut the jeans off me with scissors. (Ah, I longed for the good old days when my butt was the problem. . . .)

Speaking of my rear end, at one point I actually lost too much weight. Now you may be thinking, "I wish I'd lose my butt," but you actually can get uncomfortably thin. Remember, the butt is always greener on the other side. (And, of course, my butt returned—and it brought reinforcements.) During the brief period when I was too thin I bought myself some shorts that had the word PERFECT written across the fanny. Because for most women, a perfect butt is no butt. Until it happens to you.

Swollen ankles, giant-slipper feet, no butt—you would think the last thing I'd want is to have my picture taken. But I actually felt fortunate to be living in the same house as a professional photographer, because I wanted to document my lowest point.

We took pictures as an expression of hope. I knew I would get better, and if I didn't have pictures to prove it, no one would believe me when I told them how sick I really had been. I laid out a towel, sat down, displayed my puffy feet, and said, "I'm ready for my close-up after all, Mr. Sheinwald."

"What If Your Butt Was Gone"

If sitting in a wooden chair felt like tacks

And you found you had nothing to hold up your slacks

'Cause instead of a butt you had just a crack

Well something would have to be done

Would you call me up

Would you fall to pieces

Would you make it the topic of your doctoral thesis

Try to go out and find a prosthesis

What if your butt was gone?

• • •

Chapter 10

Mission Possible: Persistence

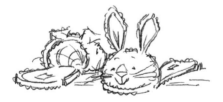

Built the Big Rubber-Band Ball—Now What?

The person who says it cannot be done should not interrupt the person doing it.

—Chinese proverb

In 2006 a man named Steve Milton and his family broke the Guinness world record for building the largest rubber-band ball. He was doing the talk-show circuit, showing footage of his creation. While it was entertaining, the advice he gave on how to accomplish something big also translates very well into a life lesson.

Here's what I got out of his advice. When you're doing something big:

1. Get help. Behind every person who ever did something difficult is a spouse or even a team of people who helped make it happen. The rubber-band-ball guy had a spouse and kids who helped him build it and who kept the enthusiasm up.
2. Do a little bit every day. Every big goal has to be broken into smaller digestible parts. Otherwise, it's like stuffing

an entire hamburger into your mouth at once—you can't even get started digesting it.

3. Put it in the garage before it gets too big. I had to think about this one—how could that possibly translate into a life lesson? I think the lesson here is to give your big goal the space it needs—and also give yourself that same space; take a break from the pursuit of your goals for a little while each day.

4. Then, the conclusion: Steve decided to use the rubber-band ball to demolish larger objects. They lifted the ball up with a crane and smashed a minivan with it. This, in an odd way, illustrates yet another point: you've got this gigantic thing—now do something with it! Help someone, inspire someone; communicate.

• • •

The Seventy-two Step Program

He who has a firm will molds the world to himself.
—Johann Wolfgang von Goethe

As any patient learns, sometimes the news is good. I went to the rheumatologist, and my tests for autoimmune disease all came back negative! I'm not sure they had ever come back negative in the entire time since my diagnosis.

I called a friend of mine to tell her the news. She and I had been hanging out just a couple weeks before, when I had predicted out loud at the dinner table: "My tests are going to come back negative."

The biggest leaps in my recovery this time came since quitting drinking diet soda, starting qigong, and going on the gluten-free/dairy-free diet. The final piece of the puzzle was my declaring and steadfastly believing that I would get the lab results to say "negative." And they did exactly that.

How to celebrate? I joked to my husband that we should go out for a big bowl of gluten and Diet Coke. I thought his face was going to shatter. Nope, I wasn't going back to my old ways; I was moving forward, and I couldn't think of a better way to celebrate being strong and healthy than to go to Philadelphia and run the Rocky steps. I did it! I ran (well, jogged) all seventy-two steps—not once, but twice!

All day long, every day, people come from all over the world to run up the Rocky steps. It means something different to everyone. For me, it was something I'd wanted to do for a long time just for fun, and because I love Rocky. But, as it turned out, running the Rocky steps was a more profound act than I realized.

After I had the strokes, I couldn't have dreamed of running stairs. In fact, I was trapped in the house because I couldn't get up and down the *one stair* that led to the outside world. Back then, the victories were smaller than testing negative for disease, like being able to wear shoes again, seeing gradual improvements in blood tests, and—finally—being able to get up and down that one stair by myself. And my celebrations were smaller, but just as meaningful: going swimming in the pool, going to the beach with a friend, going thrift shopping, or going to a concert. I always celebrate my milestones.

So what did it mean, those test results? Did it mean that I was healed? No. It meant that just for that one day, I was well. Just like someone battling an addiction, I have a condition, a tendency, that I have to keep vigil over. There are things that can trigger my condition and send me back into active disease, and every day I make choices that either aid or harm me in my recovery.

Just a couple of weeks after completing my "seventy-two-step program" (my celebratory run up the Rocky steps), a large amount of stress sent me into a two-week-long fibromyalgia attack. I recovered from that, but I had another attack a couple weeks later set off by exposure to mold. I recovered again, but shortly after that I developed Morton's neuroma, a painful foot condition that makes it very hard to even stand. I have recovered from that now, and although my tests are positive for autoimmune disease at the moment, I know it's possible to turn that around, because I did it before.

I suppose I have enough reasons to justify giving up, or sitting around feeling sorry for myself, or just resigning myself to having a drastically lowered quality of life, but I also have a lot of reasons not to. In the words of Rocky Balboa: "It's not how many times you get knocked down. It's how many times you get back up."

• • •

Conclusion: Think outside the Prescription Bottle

Mishaps are like knives that either serve us or cut us as we grasp them by the blade or the handle.

—James Russell Lowell

Have you ever had people tell you that you need to stop fighting and just accept your illness? Then they hand you a brochure on the five stages of grief. I know these people mean well, and I realize that letting go can help achieve peace of mind. But it is a personal choice, whether or not to keep fighting. For me, being asked to accept a severely diminished quality of life (I was very sick) was not acceptable. And expecting me to be on and off toxic drugs for the rest of my life, as they eat away at my bones until I end up in a wheelchair—well, that was completely unacceptable. I could not accept it. And if I had accepted it, I would still be very sick.

Sure, if I would stop asking questions and just do what the doctor tells me to, things would be a lot easier—for him. But I'm the one who has to live in this body. In general, drugs do not cure chronic diseases. They only manage the symptoms. They always have side effects, and some of those side effects are serious. One of the pamphlets that came with my prescriptions warned of increased risk of leukemia and possible fatal brain infection. If I really wanted to get better, not just manage symptoms at the risk of, well, death, I was going to have to think outside the prescription bottle. I wanted to get to the bottom of this; why was I sick?

Ultimately I realized the reason my doctors weren't giving me better answers was simple: they didn't have any. And since they didn't have any, I figured I'd look somewhere else.

If I want to succeed in business, I seek out someone who is successful. So instead of studying disease, why not study healthy people and do what they're doing? A few researchers have gone around the world looking for inherently healthy people, and they found them. According to *Never Be Sick Again*, groups in remote regions such as the Hunzas in northeastern Pakistan and the Cuenca Indians in Ecuador live to age 130 or even older, and the folks were so healthy they didn't even have words for diseases such as dementia or cancer. The "common" cold was nonexistent. None of the women got PMS.

What were they doing differently? Healthy food, vigorous exercise, fresh air, sunshine, proper sleep, low stress, close-knit community, and no pollution. Before we give the credit to good genes, check out the not-so-happy-ending: six months after the roads reached the Hunza village, followed by modern conveniences and processed foods, these legendary people began suffering from the same diseases we in the modern world suffer from.

Had I been born into a country in a remote village in some far-flung country without modern conveniences and all the trappings that come with it, I probably never would have gotten sick. Still, I don't regret anything that has happened with my health. The illness was the worst and the best thing that ever happened to me. It gave me permission to be my true self. I hated that job, hated the trailer park where I was living, and I hated wearing panty hose. I got a fresh start. Now everything in my life is there on purpose. I love my job, I love my house, I love my husband, I love my dog, and I never wear panty hose. And I have perspective. After surviving kidney failure and losing your hair, getting stuck in traffic for a couple hours on the New Jersey Turnpike is no big deal. In a way, the illness was a gift.

But I think I've learned all I need to learn from illness and I'm ready to stay well. Once, my life was consumed by being sick. Then for a while it was consumed with trying not to be sick. Finally, I found balance. I eat real food 90 percent of the time, I do qigong for ten minutes a day, I get blood tests every two months, and I get acupuncture. The rest of the time, I'm just living my life. The only thing that makes me stand out from everyone else is that I'm pursuing my dreams.

I don't expect this to happen, but if I ever get seriously ill again and find I need prescriptions, I will not refuse them. But I will also not stay on them long. Drugs do not cure chronic diseases. I'm not waiting for a miracle cure. Good food, self care, creativity, laughter—that is my miracle cure.

My hope is that something I have written here will bring you closer to finding the answers in your own quest for health, and that maybe you realize your funny bone is still intact after all.

"I Got Tremors"

(Sing to the tune of "I Got Rhythm")

I got tremors

I got numbness

I got anemia

Who could ask for anything more

I got headaches

I got nosebleeds

Kidney problems

Who could ask for anything more

Bad prognosis

I don't mind that

You will find that

I'll prove them wrong

I am stubborn

I've still got hope

I've got good friends

Who could ask for anything more

Who could ask for anything more

I got chapped lips

Toenail fungus

I've got no hair

Who could ask for anything more

But I've got choices

I've got good friends

I've got laughter

Who could ask for anything more

Who could ask for anything more

• • •

About the Author

Comical singer-songwriter Carla Ulbrich has taken her music and love of wordplay all over the United States and England. She has appeared on USA TV, the BBC, *Dr. Demento*, *The Bob and Sherrie Show*, and Sirius XM Radio. She has recorded five CDs. Ulbrich grew up in Clemson, South Carolina, and now lives in New Jersey. Visit her at www.thesingingpatient.com.